# Genetic Counseling

Papers by
Arno G. Motulsky, C. O. Carter, A. E. H.
Emery et al.

**MSS Information Corporation**
655 Madison Avenue, New York, N.Y. 10021

**Library of Congress Cataloging in Publication Data**
Main entry under title:

The Role of genetic counseling.

   1.  Genetic counseling—Addresses, essays, lectures.
I.  Motulsky, Arno G.  [DNLM: 1.  Genetic counseling—
Collected works.  QZ50 R745  1973]
RB155.R73         616'.042             73-11325
ISBN  0-8422-7150-3

# TABLE OF CONTENTS

32640

# CREDITS AND ACKNOWLEDGEMENTS

Carter, C.O., "Genetic Counselling," *The Lancet*, 1969, 1:1303-1305.

Carter, C.O., "Genetic Counselling," *Medical Clinics of North America*, 1969, 53:991-999.

Emery, A.E.H., "Genetic Counselling," *Scottish Medical Journal*, 1969, 14:335-347.

Finley, Wayne H.; and Sara C. Finley, "Inheritance," *Science*, 1967, 156:1519-1520.

Frota-Pessoa, O.; J.M. Opitz; J.G. Leroy; and K. Patau, "Counselling in Diseases Produced Either by Autosomal or X-Linked Recessive Mutations," *Acta Genetica et Statistica Medica*, 1968, 18:521-533.

Hecht, Frederick; and Everett W. Lovrien, "Genetic Diagnosis in the Newborn: A Part of Preventive Medicine," *Pediatric Clinics of North America*, 1970, 17:1039-1053.

Krmpotic, Eva; Charles Fields; and Katarina Szego, "Family Counseling," *The Chicago Medical School Quarterly*, 1970, 29:134-152.

Lynch, Henry T.; Gabriel M. Mulcahy; and Anne Krush, "Genetic Counseling (A Scientific Exhibit)," *Nebraska State Medical Journal*, 1970, 55:209-216.

Milunsky, Aubrey; John W. Littlefield; Julian N. Kanfer; Edwin H. Kolodny; Vivian E. Shih; and Leonard Atkins, "Prenatal Genetic Diagnosis," *New England Journal of Medicine*, 1970, 283:1370-1381, 1441-1447, and 1498-1504.

Motulsky, Arno G., "Human Genetics, Society, and Medicine," *The Journal of Heredity*, 1968, 59:329-336.

Nadler, Henry L., "Antenatal Detection of Hereditary Disorders," *Pediatrics*, 1968, 42:912-918.

Nadler, Henry L., "Prenatal Detection of Genetic Defects," *Journal of Pediatrics*, 1969, 74:132-143.

Sarto, Gloria E., "Prenatal Diagnosis of Genetic Disorders by Amniocentesis," *Wisconsin Medical Journal*, 1970, 69:255-260.

Taylor, Kathleen; and Robert E. Merrill, "Progress in the Delivery of Health Care," *American Journal of Diseases of Children*, 1970, 119:209-211.

Valenti, Carlo; and Tehila Kehaty, "Culture of Cells Obtained by Amniocentesis," *Journal of Laboratory and Clinical Medicine*, 1969, 73:355-358.

## PREFACE

Recent advances in genetics have made genetic counseling an important part of health care. The geneologies of various disorders have been traced and it is now possible to predict with a high degree of accuracy when a genetic anomaly is going to crop up in a family pedigree. In the case of crippling and killing disorders like Down's Syndrome, Tay-Sachs Disease or, one of a number of hemoglobinopathies, amniocentesis can be performed, thus definitely diagnosing the condition of the fetus *in utero*. Counseling can then be given on the basis of real evidence, rather than even the most carefully calculated probabilities. Amniocentesis involves some risks to the fetus; but this type of screening is feasible for cytogenetic disorders at least in women over forty, and at younger ages where the chance of cytogenetic damage seems to be great.

MSS presents in this volume the most current research on the general importance of genetic counseling, stressing the information needed to be gathered by the counselor as well as what the prospective parent needs to hear. The second section in this volume deals with prenatal genetic diagnosis, with emphasis on the specific techniques of amniocentesis and its effectiveness in diagnosis of various genetic disorders.

# The Role of Genetic Counseling

# Human Genetics,

# Society, and Medicine

Arno G. Motulsky

RECENT advances in genetic, molecular, and reproductive biology have raised the possibility of influencing human heredity more drastically than ever has been possible, thereby affecting the future course of human evolution. The fear of increasing mutation rates by radiation and chemicals as well as worry about the relaxation of selection by modern medical care have been added factors in public interest in human genetics. Most actual research activity in human genetics is carried out under medical auspices and with a medical bias. It is, therefore, likely that the initial application of the newer knowledge to man will come from this direction. It is the purpose of this paper to review the status of human genetics as it may affect society from the vantage point of a medical geneticist.

### Nature of Genetic Disease

The best understood genetic diseases are caused by single gene mutations. Such mutations may be de novo events in the germ cells of one of the parents of affected individuals. More frequently, they are transmitted to the affected patient from one or both of his parents. In autosomal dominant traits, the affected patient is a heterozygote who usually has inherited the mutant gene from one of his parents. In autosomal recessive diseases, the patient

10

is a homozygote who has inherited the mutant gene from each of his parents who both are heterozygote carriers. In many instances, recessive traits have been shown to be caused by enzymatic deficiencies. Such enzyme deficiencies are due to mutations usually affecting the structure of various enzymes. Regulatory mutations leaving enzyme structure normal have not yet been unequivocally proven in man or in any other mammal. In X-linked diseases, the mutant gene is carried on the X-chromosome and usually transmitted to affected sons by heterozygote mothers. A total of almost 1500 single gene determined traits have been identified in man. Not all of these cause disease and the proof for the nature of the claimed genetic mechanism is not solid in all these instances. The actual frequency at birth of all single gene determined traits and defects that impair health is difficult to document but probably is somewhat higher than 1 percent. This estimate implies that each specific hereditary disease is quite rare.

In many other diseases with genetic etiology, no simple Mendelian mechanism can be established, yet, family studies show an increased frequency of affected relatives. Multifactorial or polygenic inheritance is postulated implying that several unspecified genes interact with other external or internal environmental factors to produce the particular disease. The nature of some of the responsible genes has been occasionally identified. Thus, the ABO locus and the secretor locus are involved in susceptibility to peptic ulcer while the genes for the red cell traits of sickling, glucose-6-phosphate dehydrogenase deficiency, and thalassemia appear involved in protection against falciparum malaria. Many common chronic diseases such as diabetes and atherosclerosis probably have this type of inheritance. Solid advances in polygenic inheritance will require much additional work. At least 10 percent of infants at birth will be affected with diseases of this sort in later life.

Another type of genetic disease is caused by immunologically conditioned fetal—maternal incompatibility. Rh incompatibility is the best example. Mother and fetus differ in Rh type so that following leakage of some fetal red cells into the maternal circulation, the mother develops antibodies against these fetal erythrocytes. With each pregnancy, more maternal anti-Rh antibodies are stimulated, which cross the placenta and destroy the baby's Rh positive cells, with resultant hemolytic disease of the newborn. The frequency of Rh hemolytic disease at birth is 0.5 percent.

11

Finally, there is a type of genetic disease represented by the chromosomal aberrations such as various trisomies, translocations, deletions, and others. In most cases, the cellular event giving rise to the aberration presumably arises for the first time in the germ cells of one of the parents of the affected child. For instance, in trisomy 21 (mongolism or Down's syndrome) nondisjunction of a chromosomal pair (21) occurs during maternal meiosis. Familial transmission of chromosomal aberrations is much rarer. Chromosomal anomalies are relatively frequent events and are found in 0.4 percent of all live-born infants. At least 25 percent of all spontaneous miscarriages also show various chromosomal errors including triploidy. Gross cellular mishaps are, therefore, more frequent than had been suspected before the advent of cytologic technique for the visualization of mammalian chromosomes. In addition to the chromosomal aberrations that affect all body cells, a specific small deletion affecting chromosome 21 in blood-forming stem cells appears to be the primary event causing chronic granulocytic leukemia. This deletion takes place long after birth.

## Genetic Heterogeneity

Since the human organism reacts in a limited manner to various insults, different gene mutations may lead to similar clinical phenotypes. As a simple example, genetically controlled deficiencies of many different types of clotting factors will lead to bleeding disorders. Even a clinically well established entity such as hemophilia is caused by at least two different X-linked mutations, one leading to a deficiency of anti-hemophilia globulin, the other causing deficiency of plasma thromboplastin component. Many other examples could be cited. In fact, it has become a rule that careful genetic, clinical, and biochemical analyses of hereditary diseases usually shows up this type of heterogeneity.

Heterogeneity has been particularly well demonstrated with human hemoglobins. Different mutations cause various types of variant hemoglobins by substituting one amino acid for another or, more rarely by deletions of one or more amino acids of the hemoglobin polypeptide chain. About $\frac{1}{2,000}$ individuals carry an electrophoretically detectable hemoglobin abnormality, and at least 80 abnormal hemoglobins have been discovered by now. Since less than one-half of all amino acid substitutions will exhibit electrophoretic charge differences, the total number of variants probably is at least twice as high. Most hemoglobin variants appear to be of no significance for the health of their carriers and probably are selectively neutral or almost neutral. Some hemoglobins such as Hb S and probably Hb E protect their carriers from death by falciparum malaria and are relatively common in some populations. Other hemoglobin variants affect molecular stability and may be associated with red cell destruction. Others lead to chronic cyanosis, and still others cause erythrocytosis because of abnormal oxygen dissociation. Similar heterogeneity is apparent for the red cell enzyme glucose-6-phosphate dehydrogenase where 50 variants have been discovered. Depending upon the nature of the molecular lesion, some variants are innocuous; others are associated with chronic red cell destruction, and still others predispose to red cell destruction on administration of certain drugs and foods.

Enzymatic variation with no apparent health hazards has become apparent for a sizable fraction of all enzymes examined in man. Using starch gel electrophoretic techniques, various genetically determined enzyme types of different structure, but no gross difference in function, are being detected at an increasing rate. Such enzymatic variability appears to be a generalized biologic phenomenon since it also has been found in *Drosophila* and other species. As expected, many variants are quite rare, but others are fairly common in the population. The common enzyme variants qualify as polymorphisms and pose the problem of defining those evolutionary forces that have led to these high population frequencies. Chance may be the explanation in some cases. However, for many enzyme variants elevated frequencies are found in different unrelated populations and even in infrahuman species therefore requiring the postulate of selective forces, which are quite poorly understood.

Applying existing knowledge of various enzyme types to a given blood specimen, it can be shown that every individual is highly unique in his enzymatic makeup. In fact, if one combines an enzymatic profile of this type (i.e. determination of enzyme types using a battery of different enzyme markers) with a blood group and serum group profile using the various blood and serum groups, the chance that two individuals who are not identical twins will have similar enzyme, blood, or serum groups becomes negligibly small. The biologic significance of this genetic individuality promises to be of major importance for an understanding of the interaction of heredity and environment. It has already been shown that certain enzymatic variants explain

13

various drug reactions, which previously were not understood (see below). In other instances, the nature of the response to a variety of environmental agents, such as bacteria, viruses, chemicals, and stress is likely to ultimately lie in the genetically controlled biochemical makeup of man.

## Management of Genetic Disease

### Medical treatment

Understanding of the nature of a genetic abnormality often allows conventional medical curative or preventive treatment. Many examples can be given. In hemophilia, the missing anti-hemophilic globulin may be replaced. In pernicious anemia, Vitamin $B_{12}$ is not absorbed in the gut but can be replaced by periodic injections of the missing vitamin. In inborn errors of metabolism such as phenylketonuria and galactosemia the offending phenylalanine and galactose can be omitted from the diet. Removal of the spleen of patients with the red cell defect of hereditary spherocytosis allows red cells shaped in such a manner that they become trapped in the spleen to survive normally. Immunization by the Rh factor and hemolytic disease of the newborn due to the Rh factor can be completely prevented by administration of anti-Rh globulin to mothers following delivery.

More recently introduced treatments offer new hopes for some genetic diseases. The artificial kidney can maintain a productive life in patients with certain hereditary fatal kidney diseases. Kidney transplantation may offer more definite cures for such patients. The possibility of heart transplants opens the possibility for a normal life of patients with hereditary heart diseases who would die at a relatively young age.

The administration of missing enzymes by way of microcapsules implanted into the body cavities of enzyme-deficient mice and rabbits already has shown some success and is a model in approaching treatment for enzyme deficiencies in man.

### Genetic counseling

Genetic counseling is the total exchange of information regarding recurrence risks of a disease with genetic factors. Usually, parents with an affected child consult medical geneticists regarding the probability that future children will be affected. Good genetic counseling requires accurate diagnosis since, as already discussed, diseases with a similar phenotype may have a different genetic etiology. Careful evaluation of the total clinical picture and assessment of the family history are prerequisites for good genetic advice. Various laboratory tests and X rays are often required. Genetic counseling is, therefore, best provided in medical centers and many new counseling clinics are being established.

Risks will vary considerably. In autosomal dominant disorders, the recurrence risk after an affected child has been born is 50 percent. Since not all carriers of a given dominant gene will manifest the disease, the actual disease risk will often be less than 50 percent. Reversely, an affected patient who comes for counseling may often be mildly affected. Since dominant diseases often have a wide spectrum of clinical variability, their affected children have a good chance of being more severely affected. More complicated problems may arise such as the probability of a fresh mutation versus lack of gene expression as an explanation of a sporadic case with a dominant disease.

In recessive diseases, the recurrence risk is 25 percent. In recessive inheritance, the family history is frequently "negative", i.e., other sibs as well as the parent's relatives are not affected. Physicians, therefore, must recognize a given disease as a recessive trait and inform the parents that the risk of recurrence is 25 percent without being specifically asked to do so. Parents who are not told about such a risk often are understandably unhappy when another affected child is born subsequently. In X-linked recessive inheritance, there is a 50 percent risk for future boys to be affected if the mother is a heterozygous carrier, and a 50 percent risk for future girls to be carriers also. In most developmental malformations, the recurrence risks are low and often range around 5 percent. In the chromosomal disorders such as Down's syndrome recurrence risks are usually lower yet, except for the rare instances where a parent is a translocation carrier. This eventuality can be easily established by appropriate chromosomal studies.

Good genetic counseling requires knowledge about the total impact of a given disease. Parents usually are not deterred from reproduction if the disease is trivial or can be treated easily. The reaction to a fatal disorder will be different from that to one causing chronic suffering with resultant emotional, social, and financial drain on the family. Parents may be willing to take the risk of recurrence in the case of a fatal disorder, but may not be ready to incur the danger of a chronic disease. Medical geneticists usually will not tell parents whether they should or should not have more children, but will attempt to give parents the meaning of recurrence risks together with full understanding of the nature of the disease or birth defect under discussion. Different parents react quite differently to various recurrence risks and a low risk of 5 percent may appear high to some parents while a 25 percent risk may be hailed as good news by others. Parents need to be told actual risks rather than relative risks. Thus, the relative risk of recurrence of a birth defect may be many times higher than that faced by parents in the general population. If the condition is rare, the actual risk the inquiring parents face may remain rather low.

*Preventive treatment in family members at risk*

In several diseases, the diagnosis of a hereditary disease in a patient makes it mandatory that the physician examine the sibs for the presence of the disease without being directly asked for such help. Thus, in Wilson's disease, an autosomal recessive trait, there is copper infiltration of liver and brain which causes disability and death at a relatively early age. It is now possible to diagnose this disease in unaffected sibs before clinical signs are apparent. By removing the injurious copper from the body by an appropriate drug, such a sib may be spared a lethal outcome.

Similarly, in iron storage disease—an autosomal dominant trait with expression largely limited to males, appropriate measures will detect the presence of the gene in unaffected carriers. Repeated bleeding will remove the excess iron before organ damage to heart, liver, and pancreas has developed. In hereditary polyposis, an autosomal dominant trait, removal of the colon after diagnosis will prevent malignant transformation of colonic polyps which invariably occurs in untreated patients. In porphyria, an autosomal dominant trait, avoidance of barbiturate drugs may keep the trait in a latent state.

*Heterozygote detection*

The recognition that many recessive disorders are caused by enzyme deficiencies has led to the discovery of partial enzyme defects in clinically unaffected heterozygotes, i.e. parents and two-thirds of unaffected sibs. The mean enzyme level of heterozygotes is usually 50 percent of that of normal homozygotes although overlap with normals is often found in individual cases. However, whenever qualitative methods such as electrophoresis followed by histochemical visualization of the enzyme or tests based on enzyme inhibition can be devised,

16

all heterozygotes for a given defect usually can be detected. In several conditions where the exact enzyme defect is not yet known, fibroblast cultures obtained from small skin biopsies followed by various histochemical stains have been successful in detecting heterozygotes.

Heterozygote detection is of greatest practical importance in X-linked inheritance where sisters of affected patients have a 50 percent chance of being carriers; and if so affected, transmit the mutant gene to 50 percent of their sons regardless of the genotype of their husbands. Techniques exist for the identification of female carriers of several X-linked diseases. Thus, partial deficiency of anti-hemophilic globulin is found in heterozygotes of hemophilia and increased levels of the muscle enzyme creatine phosphokinase can be detected in the serum of carriers of the X-linked type of muscular dystrophy. When cell cultures are performed on heterozygote female carriers of X-linked traits, two cell populations—one normal and another abnormal—are found. In several X-linked conditions, carriers can be identified using such techniques. The ability to identify carriers is of great importance for counseling since a positive or negative diagnostic test is of considerably more help to a family than a statistical risk. The tests involved are usually fairly complicated and require many controls, and the establishment of central reference laboratories needs encouragement for only a small segment of the population now has access to these techniques.

In autosomal recessive inheritance, an unaffected sib of a patient has a $\frac{2}{3}$ chance of being a carrier but the disease can only recur in the next generation if the mate of the carrier sib also is a heterozygote carrier. Since the population frequency of heterozygotes for recessive diseases is usually less than 5 percent, the chance of future cases is very low. Thus, the ability to detect autosomal heterozygotes, is of more importance for genetic linkage and for gene frequency studies than for genetic counseling.

## Screening for Preventable Genetic Diseases

### Detection of inborn errors of metabolism

In several genetic diseases, diagnostic tests can detect the condition shortly after birth and appropriate treatment can be instituted. Phenylketonuria is the best example. This disease causes mental retardation. Dietary treatment appears to prevent the development of severe retardation although there is no full agreement whether children will be entirely normal on the diet. Laws have been passed already

17

in many states of the United States making it mandatory to test all infants at birth. Evaluation of end results has been rendered difficult by the discovery of heterogeneity in phenylketonuria. Several other conditions associated with high phenylalanine blood levels mimicking phenylketonuria have been found. Mental retardation is not necessarily seen in all of them and much additional biochemical, genetic, and clinical work is required to sort out these variants. In fact, some critics of the phenylketonuria program claim that the best results of treatment may have occurred in those patients who would not have needed dietary treatment anyway. Biochemical geneticists who have witnessed the unfolding of the remarkable heterogeneity of human proteins will not be surprised at these developments and expect the finding of heterogeneity as a general phenomenon in most genetic diseases. It is of interest that one of the hyperphenylalinemias not associated with mental retardation appears more common in patients of Mediterranean ancestry. This finding illustrates the rule that some rare genes are often concentrated in certain population groups. Detailed knowledge of a patient's ethnic origin, therefore, may be medically helpful in this context.

Already, several other inborn errors of metabolism associated with mental retardation such as galactosemia, homocystinuria, and maple syrup urine disease can be detected and serious damage possibly prevented by use of appropriate diets. Heterogeneity is already apparent in some of these defects, and additional work is required to define criteria of diagnosis and treatment in all these conditions.

The ability to identify affected patients presents many problems to society. All the diseases mentioned are quite rare, the most frequent being phenylketonuria with a frequency of at most $\frac{1}{10,000}$. The question has been raised whether sufficient technical personnel is available to run a large-scale efficient program that can maintain the required standards. Some critics have wondered whether the costs have justified the benefits of these programs, and whether the required efforts affecting a very small proportion of the population might not better be expended in other directions of genetic welfare, i.e., identification of disease in well defined high-risk groups such as the sibs of potentially curable genetic disease. Any type of screening program will have to deal with a large number of "false-positive" tests, i.e., individuals who appear abnormal on initial screening but turn out to be unaffected on detailed study. Already, some psychologic damage has been done in cases where mothers remained perturbed about the possibility of mental retardation due to phenylketonuria even though careful testing ruled out this possibility. These criticisms could be countered by pointing to the doubtless human, social, and financial benefits derived from the prevention of mental retardation in many cases.

The availability of autoanalyzers will make large-scale screening relatively simple and many other conditions will be included besides those mentioned. For instance, certain hyperlipoproteinemias are relatively common, have a simple mode of inheritance, and could be identified early in life. Dietary and drug therapy may be possible in this group of diseases and may prevent the development of atherosclerosis which occurs at a young age in these patients and may lead to premature death.

### Detection of traits predisposing to drug reactions

Certain common traits may predispose their carriers to drug reactions. Important examples include the various types of G6PD deficiency—an X-linked trait found in 10 percent of American negroes and in variable frequencies among many populations originating in tropical and subtropical areas. Trait carriers may develop blood destruction when administered a variety of commonly used oxidant drugs. Variants of the enzyme pseudocholinesterase predispose to prolonged apnea when a muscle relaxant drug commonly used during surgery —suxamethonium—is administered. One in 3,000 of the United States Caucasian population are homozygotes and at risk while the frequency among negroes is much lower. Although few hospitals have introduced routine testing for these genetic traits, such steps have been recommended and are likely to be implemented with wider use of automated methods in hospital laboratories. The population distribution of these traits is such that testing for G6PD deficiency in individuals of North European extraction and testing for pseudocholinesterase abnormalities in Afro-Americans could be omitted.

### Chromosome screening

Large-scale chromosomal screening has not yet been applied widely because of the large amount of time required for chromosomal analyses. Hopefully, in the future, automated techniques using pattern recognition devices will make it possible to apply chromosomal studies to larger populations than

19

has heretofore been possible. Such innovations are unlikely to detect many more infants with gross autosomal aberrations since such cases are picked up in many medical centers because of the presence of various congenital malformations. However, large-scale chromosomal studies are needed for an appreciation of the biologic and social significance of sex chromosomal aberrations. Fairly extensive information is already available on males with an additional X-chromosome (XXY or Klinefelter's syndrome). Such persons can be identified readily by means of buccal smears, in which a single chromatin body (like normal females but unlike normal males) is present in their exfoliated cells. The XXY karyotype is associated with infertility but also appears to have behavioral consequences. The frequency of XXY individuals is four times the expected population frequency among boys with mental retardation. An increased number of XXY individuals also have been found in mental hospitals. There is a general impression that XXY individuals tend to have a higher frequency of various character and personality disorders of the type characterized as mild psychopaths or sociopaths. These individuals often lack tenacity, may be garrulous, are unable to hold a job, and end up in various social difficulties. Large-scale testing should allow an assessment of the exact extent of this problem.

The XYY karyotype can only be recognized by full chromosomal study. No gross medical abnormality is seen in these males. However, mounting evidence suggests that the extra Y chromosome causes increased stature and abnormal asocial and probably aggressive behavior. When tall men (over 6 feet) from institutions for the criminally insane have been tested, the XYY karyotype has been frequently detected. It has been shown that XYY individuals are more likely to commit crimes against property rather than against persons, although there has been recent widespread public interest in murderers with the XYY karyotype. It has been determined that XYY individuals with a criminal record characteristically are "black sheep" and come from stable families without crime, while control criminals with a normal XY karyotype more often come from unstable families where criminal behavior in parents and sibs is found. These findings suggest strongly that the abnormal sex chromosomal constitution determines the asocial behavior of these individuals. The frequency of XYY at birth in the general population is not yet known, although estimates as high as $\frac{1}{350}$ have been made from small samples. Large-scale chromosomal screening with prospective followup of XYY persons will be necessary to define the exact behavioral risk of XYY persons. The existence of a biologically determined predisposition to criminal behavior presents difficult questions. How responsible is an XYY individual for his actions? Much discussion between lawyers, geneticists, sociologists, and criminologists will be necessary to elucidate this problem.

## Heterozygote screening and mating patterns

The increasing availability of methods allowing heterozygote detection of harmful genes has led to the suggestion of wide-scale testing of young people making the results available to prospective marriage partners. A couple with an identical harmful heterozygous gene hopefully might wish to refrain from marriage or if marriage is contracted, might refrain from reproduction. Full implementation of such a scheme would lead to complete relaxation of selection against such genes. Thus, at the present time, with each affected homozygote two harmful genes are eliminated because of early death or failure of reproduction of such individuals. If such homozygotes do not exist, the frequency of the harmful gene will slowly increase assuming that mutations continue and the heterozygote state is selectively neutral. If heterozygotes have a selective advantage (as is possible in the case of cystic fibrosis to explain the present-day frequency of 5 percent heterozygotes for this deleterious trait), failure to select against the harmful gene will cause this gene to reach a frequency of 50 percent in the population. In the case of cystic fibrosis, with a heterozygote advantage of $2\frac{1}{2}$ percent, a gene frequency of 50 percent would be reached in only 100 generations or 3,000 years. Clearly, avoidance of mating between partners carrying identical recessive genes is not necessarily the best long-term measure for every gene since the frequency of some genes would become disturbingly high.

It can be further shown that with high frequency traits, it would be necessary not only to counsel heterozygotes to avoid mating between each other but also to advise normals to marry heterozygotes occasionally. Otherwise, not enough potential marriage partners would be available to everyone in the population. Such a situation already exists in certain restricted areas of Greece, where 20 percent of the population carry the harmful blood trait, thalassemia, and another 20 percent carry the sickling trait. Genetic counseling in these areas is best carried out by encouraging marriages outside the community where such traits are much rarer. This easy solution, however, is not possible if the distribution of a common harmful gene is more uniform throughout a population. These various considerations suggest that mating schemes based on avoidance of mating of harmful gene carriers may carry certain long-term difficulties.

*Fetal diagnosis and selective abortion*

The most promising developments in genetic counseling concern techniques allowing diagnosis of various disorders of the fetus. If these techniques can be applied sufficiently early in pregnancy, therapeutic abortion of fetuses with disease could be practiced. Public attitudes towards abortion have shifted rather rapidly in recent years and several states in the United States and other countries have passed legislation allowing abortion of malformed or diseased fetuses.

Aspiration of amniotic fluid allows collection of cells of fetal origin. Sexing of the fetus can be carried out by study of chromatin bodies and abortion has been practiced when a male fetus was found in carriers of X-linked disorders such as hemophilia and muscular dystrophy. Chromosomes can be studied by culturing fetal cells and cases of translocation mongolism could be identified for selective abortion. Similarly, more complicated biochemical techniques can be applied to fetal cells following culture allowing diagnosis of a variety of disorders characterized by enzyme deficiency or by abnormal histochemical staining. As another approach, prenatal diagnosis of the adrenogenital syndrome of the fetus has been achieved by steroid assay of amniotic fluid. It may even be possible to biopsy the fetus directly using optical instruments which obtain a small skin biopsy from a visualized fetus in situ. Such tissues could then be used directly for various cytologic and biochemical methods.

What would be the consequences of selective abortion? In autosomal dominant diseases, the ability to diagnose the condition in the fetus followed by abortion would decrease the frequency of such diseases to that maintained by the mutation rate. In autosomal recessive diseases selective abortion of affected homozygotes would not change the gene frequency since at the present time most homozygotes do not reproduce. Failure to reproduce and failure to be born have identical genetical end effects. However, reproductive overcompensation for the selectively aborted homozygote could raise the gene frequency.

Selective abortion offers a means of markedly reducing the frequency of a deleterious gene from a population if abortion would not be limited to homozygote abnormals, but would include heterozygote fetuses as well. Dr. F. C. Fraser has calculated that with such a scheme, assuming two normal offspring per couple, it would require about 17 million abortions over more than one generation (30–40 years) to eliminate a gene such as that for cystic fibrosis from the United States. Even if the gene frequency could only be partially reduced by incomplete application of such measures, a reduction of gene frequency by 50 percent would reduce the autosomal recessive disease, i.e., cystic fibrosis frequency by 75 percent. The implementation of such a scheme would require heterozygote testing of all marriage partners as well as fetal testing of all offspring of heterozygote × normal and heterozygote × herteozygote matings. As long as the reason for the high frequency of the cystic fibrosis gene is unknown, there may be real danger in eliminating a gene of positive selective value. It might be argued, however, that under modern conditions, the unknown slight advantage of this gene would be of little importance. Every person carries several deleterious heterozygous genes and such schemes, therefore, could only be entertained for common recessive diseases. While such schemes are quite unacceptable under present conditions, the availability of simple methods of fetal testing and chemical methods of abortion in the future may make wider use of abortions conceivable.

In X-linked diseases, elimination of male fetuses as ascertained by nuclear sexing, whether affected or not, would have undesirable long-term effects in that more carrier females would be born who would face the problem of transmission again in the following generation. An efficient means of dealing with X-linked recessive disease would be abortion of affected males. Hopefully, the required methods to make such diagnoses will be available soon.

*Gamete and zygotic selection*

Advances in reproductive physiology have made it possible to remove rabbit blastocysts from uteri and reimplant them into recipient uteri for further development. Sexing of the zygote is possible, and embryos of the undesired sex have been discarded. This approach is less satisfactory for prevention of single gene determined disease than the development of technologies allowing separation of sperms into normal and mutant sperms with exclusion of mutant sperm from fertilization. However, no prospects

23

**Table I.** Comparison of biologic and cultural evolution. Note that the evolutionary destiny of all species was dependent upon interaction of genetic constitution and environment beyond its control. Man alone has the means to control both his environment and, to some extent, his genetic constitution.

| | Biologic evolution | Cultural evolution |
|---|---|---|
| Mediated by | Genes | Ideas |
| Rate of change | Slow | Rapid and exponential |
| Agents of change | Random variation (mutations) and selection | Usually purposeful. Directional variation and selection |
| Nature of new variant | Often harmful | Often beneficial |
| Transmission | Parents to offspring | Wide dissemination by many means |
| Nature of transmission | Simple | May be highly complex |
| Distribution in nature | All forms of life | Unique to man |
| Interaction | Man's biology requires cultural evolution | Human culture required biologic evolution to achieve the human brain |
| Complexity achieved by | Rare formation of new genes by chromosomal duplication | Frequent formation of new ideas and technologies |

for this approach are on the horizon. Separation of sperm by immunologic methods for ABO blood groups has been claimed but not confirmed. In general, sperms do not express the genotype they contain. Separation of X and Y sperms should be more readily feasible and would allow reduction of X-linked disorders if only X sperms of normal fathers married to carrier mothers were to be selected for fertilization. No males would be born with such a scheme but the longterm consequences would be an increased gene frequency of the trait in question.

### Unconventional reproductive schemes of the future

Fusion of two fertilized eggs to give rise to a mosaic individual with four parents has been achieved in mice. Fusion of as many as seven fertilized eggs have resulted in normal offspring with 14 parents! No ready reason for application of such schemes to man can be visualized unless a human society of the future would want to do away with our present two-parent system. Possibly, effects of harmful genes could be diluted in this manner.

Clonal reproduction has been sometimes discussed. In frogs it has been possible to implant intestinal tadpole cells into an enucleated egg and achieve full development into an adult frog. This experimental frog is identical in genotype to the frog from whom the intestinal cell came. The use of such a system in man would allow construction of large numbers of genetically identical individuals for specialized purposes. Scientific work, space exploration, and various other activities requiring close team work might be facilitated since genotypically identical individuals presumably could work better together. Despots of the future could abuse this method by creating powerful armies consisting of brawny soldiers of specified genotype. More frightening possibilities can be visualized. Cells from humans and primates can be hybridized in vitro. Human/primate hybrids with different degrees of contribution from each species might be created by egg fusion or by implanting somatically hybridized cells into enucleated eggs. Unlike the much discussed genetic engineering, some of the above cited developments are already technologically feasible in other species and deserve careful public debate before being applied to man.

### Selection in man

Biologists who primarily work with non-human organisms often are pessimistic about the relaxation of selection against harmful traits in man. While it is true that even individuals with handicaps

25

reproduce where animals would not, the nature of the handicap in man is a relative matter. We usually do not consider our need to wear clothes as a handicap. Yet, the mutations leading to hair loss in our species might be so considered. Myopia requiring the wearing of glasses may be viewed similarly. In fact, in the future, genetic disease such as diabetes or pernicious anemia requiring periodic injections of missing physiologic substances might not necessarily be considered as disabilities just as we do not consider the wearing of suits and glasses as a disability. Man is distinguished from all other species by his brain and by his creation of cultural innovation (Table I). Technologies can overcome many of man's genetic handicaps. Scientific technologies have only recently been applied, and the rapidity of transmission of such innovations as contrasted with the slowness of biologic evolution is likely to be able to rectify and adjust many of the problems posed by various harmful genes. Even with higher mutation rates caused by radiation and probably by chemicals, new technologies are likely to cope with most of these developments. The most acute problem facing man in the last third of the 20th century is the quantitative population explosion and not qualitative deterioration!

The nature of the relaxation of selection is sometimes overstated. In many diseases, even though life expectancies are improved by modern medical care, reproduction remains low or nonexistent. In cystic fibrosis, our most common recessive disease, reproduction of homozygotes practically does not occur. The feared deterioration of intelligence of the population because of increased reproduction rates of the less well endowed did not materialize. It could be shown that the average number of offspring of those with I.Q. 90 and below was in fact lower than that of all other individuals when married and unmarried sibs were included. In these studies, those with I.Q.'s above 116 had more children than all other groups. There is no question that selection against hereditary diseases such as diabetes has considerably relaxed. The full population dynamics of this disease, however, is not well understood. Why is it so frequent in spite of selection against affected patients until recent times?

Selection primarily exerts its effects by differential fertility and differential mortality. While differential mortality via infectious diseases has become negligible in the western world, selective mortality of birth defects and diseases with genetic components continues in our times. The remarkable phenomenon is the relative frequency of birth defects and chromo-

26

somal errors in man. We understand very little of the forces that maintain genes predisposing to these events in the population. Selective fertility may be genetically conditioned yet we remain ignorant about genetic factors affecting fertility differences. There is considerable scope for selection because of factors such as sterility and unexplained zygotic death. Since such selection may occur because of genetically determined fertility differences in the population, the wide use of birth control measures will reduce the potential for selection so that in modern societies with little variance in family size and low infantile mortality, the opportunity for selection is going to be relatively low. The above discussion makes it clear that we are largely ignorant regarding the nature of selective forces in man. It is this ignorance that should make us cautious about interfering with human reproductive and genetic process in a radical way.

## Summary

The frequency of genetic diseases is high in relation to other ills of mankind. Measures to deal with these diseases by prevention, conventional treatments, genetic counseling, and selective abortion have been considered. The various technologies and some of their difficulties have been briefly discussed. More unorthodox proposals of reproduction have been mentioned. Our ignorance regarding the forces governing selection in man and the relative nature of harmful traits in man has been emphasized. The rapidity of cultural evolution as contrasted with the slowness of biologic evolution has been stressed. It is likely that various new technologies are likely to deal with most of the problems posed by "harmful" genes without significant biologic deterioration of the human species.

This paper was presented on September 3, 1968 as the fifth Wilhelmine E. Key lecture at the annual meetings of the American Institute of Biological Sciences, held at Ohio State University, Columbus, September 3–7, 1968. The Key lecture was established by the American Genetic Association through funds bequeated to the Association by Dr. Wilhelmine E. Key for the support of lectures in human genetics.

# Genetic Counselling

C. O. CARTER, D.M., F.R.C.P.

## OBJECTIVES AND PRINCIPLES

Genetic counselling has three main functions: (1) to answer questions on recurrence risks from members of a family in which one or more cases of abnormality, thought to be genetically or part genetically determined, have already occurred; (2) to alert the medical profession to special risks that a particular pregnancy may result in a child with a genetically determined, often rare, disorder and so to make easier early diagnosis and early treatment; (3) to prevent an increase, following successful new treatment, and ultimately to reduce the proportion of children with a genetic predisposition to serious mental or physical handicap.

The demand for accurate information on recurrence risks is growing as the general public become increasingly well informed on genetics. The general principle applied by those engaged in genetic counselling is that, while the final decisions whether to take a particular risk must rest with the parents, they are entitled to the best information available on the extent of the risk. It is also necessary to put the risks into the proper perspective for the parents, both in relation to the random risk which every parent runs and also with respect to the degree of handicap which the child, if it should be affected, is likely to suffer. Experience shows that it is the relatively low recurrence risks, for example the recurrence risk of the order of 1 in 25 to normal parents following the birth of one child with cleft lip and palate, that specially need placing in the proper perspective. The implications of a 1 in 4 risk of a serious disease, for example cystic fibrosis, need little elaboration.

The decisions taken by parents after being given genetic counselling are being studied in a follow-up of some 400 patients seen by Dr. J. A. Fraser Roberts and the author at the clinic at The Hospital for Sick Children 5 to 10 years previously. It was found that where the risk was 1 in 10 or greater for a serious malformation or disease, about two thirds of the parents decided that they could not take the risk. Where the risk was less than 1 in 10, three quarters of the parents decided that they could take the risk.

## WHO SHOULD GIVE GENETIC COUNSELLING?

In some instances the general practitioner will know the recurrence risk and can himself give the risks. In others a consultant in the appropriate specialty will be well able to give the appropriate counsel. For example paediatricians know well that cystic fibrosis is a recessive disorder and the recurrence risk is 1 in 4, and haemotologists are well versed in the genetics of haemophilia. In other instances, however, the enquirer should be referred to a special genetic clinic, or where such referral is not practical, help should be sought from such a clinic. Such referral is appropriate when the genetics is not straightforward and recurrence risks are influenced by the family history, as for example in the case of the common malformations; when the patient has a rare syndrome, which could be, but is not already known to be, genetically determined; where the patient has a condition which may be inherited in more than one way, for example spondyloepiphyseal dysplasia; where special tests are available for the carrier state, for example cytogenetic tests in Down's syndrome[11] or biochemical tests for the severe X-linked form of muscular dystrophy.[8, 17]

## THE ESTIMATION OF RISKS

In assessing genetic risks the two essentials are the taking of an accurate family tree, with verification, from hospital records or other sources, of the medical history of possibly affected members; and an exact diagnosis.[3, 4] It is sometimes possible to be reasonably sure of the pattern of inheritance on the basis of the family history alone. This is exceptional, however, and most often the patient who is the reason for the enquiry is the only one affected in the family. Genetic counselling then depends essentially on the diagnosis and the counsellor's knowledge of the way in which that particular condition is inherited or, if no simple genetic determination is involved, the counsellor's knowledge of the empirical recurrence risks for that particular condition.

In practice it is usually possible, where the exact risk is not known, to give the enquirer the right order of risk. Risks fall into three groups: those in which the recurrence risk is little or no more than the random risk for all births in the population; those in which there is a high risk of recurrence of the order of 1 in 10 or more; and those in which there is a moderate risk of recurrence, of the order of less than 1 in 10 and usually less than 1 in 20.

The over-all accuracy of the estimation of risks of recurrence is shown by the findings of the follow-up at The Hospital for Sick Children, referred to above and summarised in Table 1.

In this table high risk cases include all those in which the risk was 1 in 10 or greater (most often 1 in 4); low risk includes those in which it was less than 1 in 10 (usually less than 1 in 20). The observed recurrence in the high risk group is 1 in 4½ and in the low risk group 1 in 50; this is satisfactorily close to prediction.

**Table 1.** *Children Born Subsequent to Counselling*

|  | TOTAL | AFFECTED LIKE INDEX PATIENT | PROPORTION |
|---|---|---|---|
| High risk (129) | 62 | 14 | 1 in 4½ |
| Low risk (177) | 154 | 3 | 1 in 50 |

## ONLY RANDOM RISKS OF RECURRENCE

In the first group with little or no more than the random risk in the general population the counsellor can be reassuring, though he cannot give the guarantee of normality in any subsequent pregnancy for which some enquirers ask. Conditions that fall into this group include those in which there is some environmental cause of the patient's handicap and this cause is not likely to operate in a subsequent pregnancy. Rubella, toxoplasmosis, and thalidomide embryopathy are examples. This group also includes, however, a substantial number of instances of conditions that are genetically determined, but in which the patient has been affected as a result of a fresh mutation. For example the great majority of children with chromosome abnormalities, including those with Down's syndrome, are affected as a result of fresh mutations.[8] A large majority of children affected by severe dominant conditions which substantially reduce biological fitness are affected as a result of fresh mutations; examples are classical achondroplasia and tuberous sclerosis. In both instances, provided that the genetic anomaly always causes clinical manifestations and neither parents nor other near relatives are affected, the recurrence is little increased over the random risk. At present the best estimates of the recurrence risk after a sporadic case of Down's syndrome, in which there is regular G trisomy and both parents are chromosomally normal, is twice the random risk for a mother of that age.[5, 11] Similarly, though no large scale series are available for the dominant condition tuberous sclerosis (epiloia), it is certainly rare to find a second affected child in a sibship where neither parent has any manifestation of the condition.

Where recurrence does occur after sporadic cases of regularly dominant conditions, it may well be that the mutation has occurred not in gamete formation, but further back in the germ cell line, so that a portion of the gonad of one or the other parent consists of cells with the mutation. Fortunately this appears to be an unusual phenomenon.

## HIGH RISK CONDITIONS

There are three sources of high risks: a few instances of chromosome anomalies where a balanced anomaly is present in one or the other parent; many instances of conditions determined by mutant genes of large effect; a few instances of conditions due to more complex inheritance.

CHROMOSOME ANOMALIES. The high or relatively high risk situation with chromosome anomalies is exemplified by the perhaps 1 per cent of

30

instances of Down's syndrome where the child has 46 chromosomes with a D/G translocation, and one or the other parent has 45 chromosomes with the same translocation. The empirical risk figures are not yet established,[5] and it will need prospective studies to determine them with accuracy, but where the mother has such a translocation the recurrence risk of a liveborn child with Down's syndrome is of the order of 1 in 5 to 1 in 10; where the father has the translocation, it is probably less than 1 in 20. Where a G/G translocation is present the risk is probably somewhat higher. If the child has regular G trisomy and one parent has mosaicism with one cell line having G trisomy, the recurrence risk cannot be accurately assessed and is likely to be raised, but is probably less than 1 in 10. Chromosome studies are advisable especially if the mother was under 30 years of age when the patient was born. There is a special case for chromosome studies before giving counsel when the child is affected by a structural anomaly, for example the cri-du-chat syndrome due to a deletion of the short arm of a B chromosome, since these not uncommonly occur from a balanced translocation in one or the other parent.

An important new development for genetic counselling is the development of intrauterine diagnosis of chromosome anomalies by suprapubic amniocentesis at about the fourteenth week of pregnancy followed by culture of the foetal cells in the amniotic fluid.[12] At present the procedure appears safe and a good proportion of cultures succeed. Parents, if they wish to take the risk of a further pregnancy, may be offered this test, and if the foetus is shown to have an unbalanced chromosomal abnormality they may be offered a termination. Instances of the detection of both chromosomally normal and abnormal foetuses have already been reported in pregnancies in mothers with D/G translocations.[12, 16]

It is likely that this procedure, if proved safe, will be extended to patients with increased, but relatively low, risks—for example, to all pregnant women over the age of 40 years, when the risk of G trisomy alone is more than 1 per cent.

CONDITIONS DUE TO MUTANT GENES OF LARGE EFFECT. The general principles of genetic counselling for conditions due to mutant genes of large effect are given below: exact diagnosis is important and it is also important to remember that one clinical condition may be inherited in more than one way; for example, severe childhood muscular dystrophy may be either X-linked or recessive.

With dominant conditions, manifest in individuals heterozygous for the mutant gene concerned, the essential risk is the 1 in 2 risk to the offspring of the unaffected members of the family or to the sibs of the first affected member in the family. Two normal parents with a son with classical achondroplasia may as mentioned above be told that the risk of achondroplasia in their own further children is small, that the risk to their grandchildren born to any normal children they may have is also small, but that the risk to the children of their affected son is 1 in 2. Difficulties in counselling with dominant conditions may come from the variability of manifestation in those heterozygous for the gene, or from the late onset of the clinical manifestation. Where heterozygotes always show at least some manifestation, the need is only to make sure that such minor manifestations are not missed. For example five or more café-au-lait patches of skin may be the only manifestation of the gene responsible for von Recklinghausen's disease.

Where the condition is not truly dominant in the sense that heterozygotes may sometimes show no manifestation at all, counselling must be amended accordingly. Patients with bilateral retinoblastoma are heterozygotes for a mutant gene, but there are also individuals who must be heterozygotes, since they have transmitted the gene, but have no clinical manifestations themselves. Fortunately this is unusual, but it does mean that normal parents cannot be told that it is most unlikely they will have another affected child, and normal sibs of a patient cannot be told that they are most unlikely to transmit the condition.

With dominant conditions of late onset, for example, Huntington's chorea, it is usually impossible to decide at, say, age 20 years, whether a particular man or woman genetically at risk is or is not a heterozygote at the time they marry. It is reasonable to hope, however, that it may prove possible before long to find biochemical tests for heterozygotes for such mutant genes which will enable them to be picked up even though there is no clinical manifestation. For example, heterozygotes for the mutant gene responsible for variegate porphyria may be without clinical manifestation, but may be detected in many instances by increased protoporphyrin in stools.[7] Where the biochemical abnormality proves to be one that may be detected in amniotic cells, the procedure of amniocentesis will be of great value for patients with severe dominant conditions, who are willing to accept an offer of termination where the foetus proves to be a heterozygote.

With recessive conditions, manifest in individuals homozygous for the mutant gene concerned, the essential risk is the 1 in 4 risk to any subsequent child of the parents, where both parents are unaffected. In the rare instances where one parent, as well as the patient, is affected, the risk to any further child is 1 in 2. In the very rare instance where a child and both parents are affected by a recessive condition, any further child will be affected. Such marriages of individuals homozygous for the same recessive gene only occur in practice among the deaf and the blind. With recessive conditions the risks to members of the family other than sibs is usually small. The commonest serious recessive condition in Europeans is cystic fibrosis, which has a frequency at birth of about 1 in 2000, corresponding to a gene frequency at birth of a little less than 1 in 40. Even here the risk to the children of surviving patients is about 1 in 40, and the risk to the children of the patients' brothers and sisters is about 1 in 120, provided that cousin marriage is avoided.

Genetic counselling is made more precise with recessive conditions once the heterozygous carriers of the mutant gene are detected. This is in most cases impossible until the biochemical defect has been discovered. There is, however, an ever-increasing list of conditions for which the basic defect has been found. With rare conditions such tests are worthwhile for members of the family in which a patient has already been born. With common conditions, once a quick and reliable test has been found, it will be worthwhile to screen populations, such as children at school medical examinations, and warning the known heterozygotes of the risks to their children if they should intermarry. Tests for the hetero-zygotes are already available for cystic fibrosis,[6] though these are too slow and costly as yet for use as routine screening procedures. Where it is known that two heterozygotes for the same mutant gene have married, amniocentesis again offers the hope of intrauterine detection of the homo-zygotes, with the opportunity to offer the parents a termination when-ever the biochemical deficiency is detectable in amniotic cells. The simpler and more rapid test, by the effect of plasma from heterozygotes on ciliary activity,[1, 15] is not yet fully reliable, but may well be improved.

Amniocentesis will in the future be a valuable supplement to genetic counselling in those recessive conditions where the biochemical defect is demonstrated in amniotic cells, particularly where the heterozygotes can be distinguished from the homozygotes.

With X-linked conditions the essential risk is the 1 in 2 risk of the condition to the sons of known heterozygous women and the 1 in 2 risk of daughters of such women being heterozygotes. A woman is almost always a heterozygote if she has had an affected son and any other male relative is also affected. Thus a woman with two affected sons, a woman with an affected son and an affected brother, and a woman with an af-fected son whose sister also has an affected son, are all very likely to be carriers on genetic grounds. A woman whose father was affected is also almost certainly a carrier. Often, however, the family history gives only a risk that a woman is a heterozygote; for example, the 1 in 2 risk that a daughter of a known heterozygous carrier is a carrier, or the less precise risk that a woman with an affected son, but no other male relative af-fected, is a carrier. In the latter instance the risk may be estimated more precisely from the information available on other members of the family, especially the number of unaffected sons and brothers the woman has.[8, 14] With X-linked conditions, however, it is especially important to find methods of detecting carriers. Most men and women who are hetero-zygous for a mutant gene which causes a serious condition in homozy-gotes will be lucky enough to marry a spouse who is not a heterozygote for the same mutant gene. In contrast, all women who are heterozygous for X-linked genes are at risk of having affected sons, and this is indepen-dent of the husband's genotype.

It is, fortunately, often possible to detect women heterozygous for X-linked mutant genes by relatively simple clinical tests, before the bio-chemical deficiency in the affected males has been discovered. The ex-planation probably lies in the inactivation of one X chromosome in women, and the fact that the active X chromosome in some cells is that with the mutant gene. Examples of such simple clinical tests[8] are: the urine concentration test in women heterozygous for the gene for the X-linked form of nephrogenic diabetes insipidus; serum creatine kinase levels in the case of the two X-linked forms of muscular dystrophy;[17] factor IX levels in haemophilia B; and metachromatic granules in fibro-blast culture in the case of X linked mucopolysaccharidosis.[6] While in some instances the distinction between heterozygous carriers and normal women is absolute, in others there is overlap between the distribution of values on the test for the two types of women. Nevertheless, if both distributions are established it is possible to estimate the relative probabilities of a particular woman belonging to one type or the other and to combine this with the genetic probability, based on the pedigree, to give a total probability that a woman is or is not a carrier.[8, 17] For this kind of comparison, however, it is best that tests on patients and controls should all be done in the same laboratory.

Amniocentesis will be of great value with X-linked conditions if the biochemical abnormality is known and is demonstrable in amniotic cells. An example of successful use of the procedure has already been reported with the X-linked hyperuricaemia syndrome.[10] Looking further ahead when couples can choose the sex of their children, affected males may safely have as many sons as they wish without fear of further transmission of the gene concerned.

An admirably complete list of conditions determined by mutant genes is given with selected references by McKusick.[13] A shorter list of conditions with onset in childhood is given by Blyth and Carter.[2]

## MODERATE RISKS AND COMMON CONDITIONS

Few conditions that are both serious and common are determined by a simple genetic mechanism. A few conditions due to chromosomal anomalies have frequencies of between 1 and 2 per thousand births of the appropriate sex — for example Down's, Klinefelter's, and the triple X syndromes. A few recessive conditions have such frequencies in special areas, for example sickle-cell anaemia, thalassaemia and glucose-6-phosphate dehydrogenase deficiency. In most instances, however, where a common condition has a considerable element of genetic causation, this genetic element is polygenic depending on allelism at several gene loci.[3, 9] In almost all instances this polygenic predisposition will interact with environmental factors. Such in part genetically determined conditions include common congenital malformations such as spina bifida, anencephaly, cleft lip and palate, congenital dislocation of the hip, club foot, and pyloric stenosis, and common diseases such as schizophrenia, diabetes mellitus, and ischaemic heart disease.

Genetic counselling for such conditions depends on establishing empirical risks. Such risks are estimated by large-scale family studies on index patients drawn, if possible, from the same population as the family asking for counselling. In general, with polygenic inheritance, the higher the frequency of the condition in the population, the higher the recurrence risk. This does not necessarily apply, however, since the relative contributions of the genetic and environmental elements in causation may vary from one population to another. It is also important to note that with this type of genetic determination the recurrence risk will vary from one family to another. With a recessive condition, for example cystic fibrosis of the pancreas, the recurrence risk remains 1 in 4 whether the parents have had one, two, or three affected children. With moderate risk conditions depending on polygenic inheritance, the recurrence risk will be modified by the previous experience of the family. The risk will be higher where two affected children have already been born, or where an affected parent has already had one affected child. The risk is also likely to be higher when the child belongs to the less commonly affected sex. Apart from some such special situations, however, the recurrence risks with these common conditions are usually only moderate. They are not such as will deter most parents from having further children, but they may well be important in alerting the medical services to a special risk to a particular unborn child.

An important feature of genetic counselling for these common conditions is to recognise rare forms of the condition which are more simply inherited, and which may carry a different recurrence risk from the main group. For example cleft lip, with or without cleft palate, may occur with mucous pits of the lower lip in the rare Van de Woude's syndrome, which is a regular dominant. Cleft lip and palate may also occur as one manifestation of D trisomy (Patau's syndrome).

Approximate empirical risk figures for some common paediatric conditions are summarised below. A fuller account is given by Carter.[3]

*Cleft lip with or without cleft palate.* If both parents are normal, risk for sibs or children of index patients is 1 in 25; if one parent and one child are affected, risk to subsequent sibs is about 1 in 8.

*Cleft palate, median and uncomplicated.* Undoubtedly of heterogeneous aetiology, risk to subsequent sibs when parents are normal is 1 in 50; when parents are normal but another relative is affected, 1 in 10; when one parent as well as the patient is affected, 1 in 6; risk to children 1 in 50.

*Congenital malformations of the heart.* Aetiology heterogeneous, but risks to sibs mostly 1 in 25 to 1 in 30, but only 1 to 2 per cent for patent ductus arteriosus.

*Myelocoele, meningocoele, encephalocoele, and anencephaly.* Risk to sibs of one or other form of neural tube malformation varies with the population frequency at birth from 1 in 15 to 1 in 30. Risk after two malformed children is about 1 in 8.

*Congenital dislocation of the hip.* Risk to female sibs or children of girl patients is 1 in 15 and to male relatives of girl patients 1 in 100; higher risks for relatives of male patients.

*Pyloric stenosis.* For male patients, the risk to sons and brothers is 1 in 20, to daughters and sisters 1 in 40; for female index patients, the risk to sons 1 in 5, to brothers 1 in 10, to daughters 1 in 15, and to sisters 1 in 25.

*Talipes equinovarus.* Risk to sibs and children 1 in 50.

*Scoliosis (idiopathic).* Risk to relatives of cases with early onset 1 in 30 to 1 in 50; risk to sibs of adolescent female cases about 1 in 10 for sisters and 1 in 50 for brothers.

*Diabetes mellitus of early onset.* Risk to sibs of early onset of disease is 1 in 20.

*Infantile autism.* Heterogeneous, but over-all risk to sibs is about 1 in 50.

*Nonspecific severe mental retardation.* Heterogeneous group, but over-all risk of recurrence is 1 in 20.

# REFERENCES

1. Besley, G. T. N., Patrick, A. D., and Norman, A. P.: Inhibition of the mobility of gill cilia of Dreissensia by plasma of cystic fibrosis patients and their parents. J. Med. Genet., in press.
2. Blyth, H., and Carter, C. O.: A guide to genetic prognosis in paediatrics, Devel. Med. Child Neurol., Suppl. 18, 1969.
3. Carter, C. O.: Genetics of common disorders. Brit. Med. Bull., 25:52, 1969.
4. Carter, C. O.: Genetic counselling for the common malformations. In Motulsky, A. G., ed.: Counselling and Prognosis in Medicial Genetics. New York, Hoeber Medical Division, Harper & Row, in press.
5. Carter, C. O., and Evans, K. A.: Risk of parents who have had one child with Down's syndrome (mongolism) having another child similarly affected. Lancet, 2:785, 1961.
6. Danes, B. S., and Bearn, A. G.: A genetic marker in cystic fibrosis of the pancreas. Lancet, 1:1061, 1968.
7. Dean, C.: The porphyrias. Brit. Med. Bull., 25:48, 1969.
8. Emery, A. E. H., and Morton, R.: Genetic counselling in X-linked disorders. Acta Genet. Basel, 8:534, 1969.
9. Falconer, D. S.: The inheritance of liability to certain diseases estimated from incidence among relatives. Ann. Hum. Genet., 29:51, 1965.
10. Fujimoto, W. Y., Seegmuller, O. E., Uhlendorf, B. W., and Jacobson, C. B.: Biochemical diagnosis of an X-linked disease in utero. Lancet, 2:511, 1968.
11. Hamerton, J. L., Briggs, S. M., Giannelli, P., and Carter, C. O.: Chromosome studies in detection of parents with a high risk of a second child with Down's syndrome. Lancet, 2:788, 1961.
12. Jacobson, C. B., and Barter, R. H.: Intrauterine diagnosis and management of genetic defects. Amer. J. Obstet. Gynec., 99:796, 1967.
13. McKusick, V. A.: Mendelian Inheritance in Man: Catalogs of Autosomal Dominant, Autosomal Recessive and X-Linked Phenotypes. Baltimore, Johns Hopkins Press, 1966.
14. Murphy, E. A.: The rationale of genetic counselling. J. Pediat., 72:121, 1968.
15. Spock, A., Heick, H. M. C., Cress, H., and Logan, W. S.: Abnormal serum factor in patients with cystic fibrosis of the pancreas. Pediat. Res., 1:173, 1967.
16. Valenti, C., Schutta, E. S., and Kehaty, T.: Prenatal diagnosis of Down's syndrome. Lancet, 2:220, 1968.
17. Wilson, K. M., Evans, K. A., and Carter, C. O.: Creatine kinase levels in women who carry genes for three types of muscular dystrophy. Brit. Med. J., 1:750, 1965.

M.R.C. Clinical Genetics Unit
Institute of Child Health
30 Guilford Street
London W.C.1, England

# GENETIC COUNSELLING

## C. O. CARTER

THE three objectives of genetic counselling are: firstly, to answer parents' questions on risks of recurrence in another child, when a member of the family has some malformation or disease which might be genetically determined; secondly, to draw attention to a special risk that a particular child may be born with a genetically determined (often rare) disease, so that diagnosis may be made and treatment started promptly; thirdly, to prevent an increase, following new treatments, in the frequency of children born genetically predisposed to serious handicap, and ultimately to reduce the proportion of children so born to well below the frequency determined by the natural balance between mutation and selection.

The demand from parents for information on genetic risks is growing as they increasingly plan, and so feel responsible for, the birth of each child, and as they become increasingly knowledgeable about genetics. They are entitled to be told what the risks are, in so far as they are known, and to have the risk put into proper perspective in relation both to the possible severity of the condition and to the random risk for any parental couple. Experience shows that parents normally make sensible decisions on whether or not to plan further children once they have been told what are the risks.

The need to alert the medical profession to special risk increases as treatments become available for genetically or partly genetically determined disorders. Such treatments are often effective only if they are begun early. These treatments may be medical, as with phenylketonuria, galactosæmia, and essential hypercholesterolæmia, or surgical, as with Hirschsprung's disease, pyloric stenosis, meconium ileus associated with cystic fibrosis of the pancreas, and multiple polyposis of the colon.

Conditions that are wholly or partly genetically determined are becoming increasingly prominent as public-health problems, because of the success of the environmental-health services in reducing the incidence of environmentally determined disease. New techniques for the detection of heterozygous carriers for the mutant genes responsible for autosomal recessive and X-linked recessive diseases offer new hopes of preventing such diseases by counselling. New techniques for detecting chromosome anomalies, and some inborn errors of metabolism, early in pregnancy in cells obtained by amniocentesis, or perhaps even earlier in pregnancy by chorion biopsy, offer the prospect of reducing the frequency at birth of such anomalies. This will be achieved by the offer of a termination of the pregnancy when the fetus is demonstrably abnormal.

### Assessment of Risks

Accurate assessment of genetic risk depends firstly on an accurate diagnosis, secondly on a good family history with verification of relevant medical information from hospital or other records, and thirdly on knowledge of the way in which the particular condition is inherited.

Occasionally the family history by itself will leave little doubt about the way in which the condition is inherited, but in most cases prognosis depends on the two other guides—accurate diagnosis and knowledge of the inheritance of the condition based on the families of many index patients. Accuracy of diagnosis is of special importance in genetic counselling, in that many conditions which were regarded, not unreasonably, as clinical entities, proved on genetic analysis to be compounded of different entities with different genetic determination. The X-linked Hunter's and the autosomal recessive Hurler's forms of mucopolysaccharidosis (gargoylism) are examples.[1] So are the X-linked and the recessive forms of severe childhood muscular dystrophy,[2][3] and the dominant, recessive, and X-linked forms of spondylo-epiphyseal dysplasia.[4] The genetic counsellor should be well versed in the clinical specialty into which the patient's condition fits, as well as having a good understanding of genetics.

In practice, risks fall into three groups: those in which the risk of recurrence is little or no more than the random risk of the particular condition in any child; those in which there is a high risk of recurrence (1 in 10 or higher); and those in which there is a moderate risk of recurrence, considerably greater than the random risk, but better than 1 in 10, and usually better than 1 in 20.[5] It is often convenient to combine the random and moderate risks into a " low "-risk category.

### Random Risks

Random risks apply when there is an environmental cause of a patient's handicap which is not likely to recur in a later pregnancy—for example, maternal rubella or toxoplasmosis. Near-random risks of recurrence in later sibs also apply in many instances where the patient's anomaly is genetically determined, but as a result of a fresh chromosomal or gene mutation. The great majority of children with syndromes due to chromosome anomalies (including Down's syndrome) have parents who appear to be chromosomally normal. Most children affected by severe dominant conditions will be affected by fresh mutations.

After a sporadic case of Down's syndrome, where chromosome tests show that the child has regular G trisomy and both parents are chromosomally normal, the empirical risk to later sibs, based on a large series, appears to be about double the random risk for a mother of that age.[6][7] After sporadic cases of dominant conditions, such as achondroplasia or tuberous sclerosis, the empirical recurrence risk to later sibs appears, in the small series available, to be low. Some dominant conditions show variable manifestation: it is important, for instance, to make sure that neither parent of a child with tuberous sclerosis has a slight degree of adenoma sebaceum. In the rare instances where there is a recurrence after a sporadic case of a regularly dominant condition it is probable that the mutation has occurred earlier in the cell-line than gamete formation, so that a portion of the gonad contains a fresh mutation.

### High-risk Conditions

In most instances where there is a high risk of recurrence the patient has a condition due to a mutant gene of large effect which is not a new mutation. There are also, however, a minority of cases where a condition due to a chromosome anomaly carries a high risk of recurrence. In these cases the child is affected by a structural chromosomal anomaly, and the anomaly is present in balanced form in one or other parent. For example, where a mother has a D/G translocation the risk of recurrence of Down's syndrome in a later pregnancy is of the order of 1 in 5 to 1 in 10.[8] Where the father has the translocation the risk is probably less than 1 in 20. Where a child and parent have a G/G translocation the risk is probably somewhat higher. There is a special need for chromosome studies for genetic counselling for conditions which are always due to a structural chromosome anomaly—for example, the cri du chat syndrome due to a deletion of a short arm of a B chromosome. An important recent advance for genetic counselling for chromosome anomalies is the culture of embryonic cells obtained by amniocentesis at the 14th–16th week after conception.[9][10] Several examples have now been reported where a mother who has had a child with Down's syndrome, and has herself a D/G translocation, has embarked on another pregnancy, and the fetus has been screened in this way.

These account for the majority of high-risk situations. The general principles of genetic counselling here may be summarised as follows: with dominant conditions there is a 1-in-2 risk to the children of affected members of the family, but little risk to later sibs of the first sporadic case in the family; with recessive conditions there is a 1-in-4 risk to later sibs of affected children, but little risk to anyone else in the family, even to the children of index patients; with X-linked conditions the essential risk is the 1-in-2 risk to the sons of known heterozygous carrier women.

The difficulties in counselling for dominant conditions arise from the variability of manifestation shown by many of them, and, sometimes, from the late onset of clinical manifestations. Where a family member shows even very slight manifestations he must be assumed to be a heterozygote for the gene concerned and capable of transmitting it. Early cataract, visible on slit-lamp examination, may be the first indication of dystrophia myotonica. Five or more café-au-lait spots more than 1·5 cm. in diameter may be the only sign of neuro-fibromatosis.[11] Where heterozygotes may in some instances show no clinical manifestation whatsoever genetic advice must be modified accordingly. Patients who are heterozygous for the gene for retinoblastoma may transmit without themselves being affected. This is fortunately unusual, but normal parents of a sporadic case of bilateral retinoblastoma cannot be told that there is little risk of recurrence in later sibs. Small series suggest, however, that the recurrence risk is less than 1 in 10. With Huntington's chorea, since the onset is usually in the fourth and fifth decade, it is at present unfortunately not possible in most instances to distinguish between the young members of the family who are and are not likely to transmit the condition at the time when they wish to marry. Biochemical tests for heterozygotes would be of great value. For example, many heterozygotes for the gene for variegate porphyria, who are without clinical manifestation, may be detected by the increased proto-porphyrins in their stools.[12]

With recessive conditions the risks to relatives, other than sibs, is usually small and may be estimated from the gene frequency. Patients with phenylketonuria treated early are now surviving without severe mental handicap. These patients must transmit the gene, but, married to an unrelated individual, the chance that the spouse will also transmit the gene is the same as the gene frequency. In south-east England and much of the United States this gene frequency is probably of the order of 1 in 150; in Eire it is perhaps 1 in 70. Similarly, children with cystic fibrosis of the pancreas, the commonest recessive

40

disorder in northern and central Europe, arc now surviving into adult life. Although the men with this condition are probably all sterile, the women are fertile, and the risk to their children is, in south-east England, of the order of 1 in 45. The risks to nephews and nieces of patients is one-third that of the risk to children, since the likelihood of an unaffected sib of a patient being a heterozygote for the mutant gene is 2 in 3. Genetic counselling becomes more precise for recessive conditions once tests for the heterozygous carriers become available. This is usually not until the basic biochemical defect has been found. When a test is available it is desirable to test those genetically at risk and their prospective spouses. Where a recessive condition is a real public-health problem, owing perhaps to a heterozygote advantage, there is a case for screening all children for the carrier state. Where the biochemical defect in a recessive condition is demonstrable in fibroblast culture, amniocentesis, followed by the offer of termination if the fetus is affected, will provide a valuable supplement to genetic counselling. Amniocentesis has already been used in relation to glycogen-storage disease, galactosæmia, and maple-syrup urine disease.[10]

In X-linked conditions genetic counselling depends on estimating the probability that a woman in a family at risk is or is not a carrier. In contrast to carriers of genes for autosomal recessive conditions, all women heterozygous for X-linked conditions have a 1-in-2 risk of having affected sons, and this is independent of the husband's genotype. A woman is almost certainly a heterozygote if she has an affected son and another male relative is affected. A woman with two sons, or a son and a brother, or a son and a sister's son, affected may for practical purposes be assumed to be a carrier. The daughter of an affected man is always a carrier. A woman with an affected son but no other male relative affected may be a carrier, but she may also, if her son is affected as a result of a fresh mutation, be genetically normal. The risk of such a woman being a carrier may be estimated on the assumption of equal mutation-rates in sperms and ova, from the number of her unaffected sons and brothers.[13][14] Genetic counselling, however, is made much more precise by special tests for the carrier state. Fortunately, because of the random inactivation of one X chromosome in women which will lead to some cells in most tissues having the X chromosome with the mutant gene active, it is often possible to detect some, at least, of the carriers before the precise biochemical defect in affected males has been found. Examples are: the urine-concentration test in X-linked nephrogenic diabetes insipidus; serum-creatine-kinase levels in the two X-linked forms of muscular dystrophy; factor-IX levels in hæmophilia B; metachromatic granules in fibroblast culture in the

41

X-linked mucopolysaccharidosis.[14] The distinction, by such tests, between normal and heterozygous women is often not absolute, but it is nevertheless possible to estimate, from the distribution curve of test results in the two classes of women, the relative probability that a particular woman is normal or a carrier. This biochemical probability may be combined with the genetic probability to give a useful total probability that a woman at risk is a carrier. Amniocentesis again will be a help to genetic counselling where the biochemical abnormality is demonstrable in fibroblast culture, as with the Lesch-Nyham type of hyperuricæmia.[15]

*Multifactorial Traits*

In a minority of instances of multifactorial traits with a polygenic predisposition the recurrence risk may be more than 1 in 10. These are mostly instances in which two children are already affected,[16] [17] or a parent and child are affected.

## Moderate Risks and Common Conditions

Knowledge of moderate risk of recurrence (less than 1 in 10, but substantially more than the random risk in the general population) is perhaps of more importance in alerting the family's medical practitioner to the special risk than as an indication for family limitation. Such moderate-risk situations are found in a minority of chromosome anomalies (for example, where the father has a balanced D/G translocation) and in a minority of conditions due to a mutant gene of large effect (for example, the children of a woman with cystic fibrosis). The great majority of moderate-risk situations, however, occur when the patient has a common malformation or disease for which the genetic predisposition is polygenic.

Genetic counselling for such conditions depends essentially on establishing empiric-risk figures based on large-scale family studies of patients drawn from the same population as the patient.[17] In general, with such conditions the higher the population incidence the higher the recurrence risk. One would expect the recurrence risk after a neural-tube malformation to be lower in a low-incidence area such as Japan than in South Wales where it is about 6%. The recurrence risk may vary with the sex of the index patient, as with pyloric stenosis and congenital dislocation of the hip. The risk will be influenced by the presence of affected near relatives of the patient. Accurate diagnosis is again important. Some rare forms of a common condition, for example, may be determined by a mutant gene of large effect. Cleft lip and palate when associated with mucous pits of the lower lip (Van de Woude's syndrome) is a dominant condition; cleft lip and palate may occur in D trisomy (Patau's syndrome).

With moderate-risk situations it is especially important to put the risk into proper perspective for the parents. A 1-in-25 risk of cleft-lip malformation after normal parents have had one such child must be seen in the perspective that about 1 in 40 of all children at birth in White populations have a serious congenital malformation.[18] In general, those concerned with genetic counselling leave decisions to the parents, but it is the author's practice, when risks are of 1 in 20 or less, to volunteer that " in your place I would not take a risk of this order too seriously ".

### REFERENCES

1. McKusick, V. A. Heritable Disorders of Connective Tissue. Saint Louis, 1966.
2. Stevenson, A. C. *Ann. Eugen.* 1953, **18**, 50.
3. Blyth, H., Pugh, R. *Ann. hum. Genet.* 1959, **23**, 127.
4. Carter, C. O., Sutcliffe, J. Symposium Ossium. Edinburgh (in the press).
5. Roberts, J. A. F. Introduction to Medical Genetics; p. 254. London, 1963.
6. Carter, C. O., Evans, K. A. *Lancet*, 1961, ii, 785.
7. Hamerton, J. L., Briggs, S. M., Gianelli, F., Carter, C. O. *ibid.* p. 788.
8. Hamerton, J. *Cytogenetics*, 1968, **7**, 260.
9. Jacobson, G. B., Barter, R. H. *Am. J. Obstet. Gynec.* 1967, **99**, 796.
10. Nadler, H. L. *J. Pediat.* 1969, **24**, 132.
11. Crowe, F. W., Schull, W. J., Neel, J. V. Multiple Neurofibromatosis, p. 25 Springfield, Illinois, 1956.
12. Dean, G. *Br. med. Bull.* 1969, **25**, 48.
13. Murphy, E. A. *J. Pediat.* 1968, **72**, 121.
14. Emery, A. E. H., Morton, R. *Acta genet. Statist. med.* 1969, **18**, 534.
15. Fujimoto, W. Y., Seegmuller, J. E., Uhlendorf, B. W., Jacobson, C. B. *Lancet*, 1968, ii, 511.
16. Carter, C. O., Roberts, J. A. F. *Lancet*, 1967, i, 306.
17. Carter, C. O. *in* Counselling and Prognosis in Medical Genetics (edited by A. G. Motulsky). New York (in the press).
18. Roberts, J. A. F. Introduction to Medical Genetics; p. 265, London, 1963.

# GENETIC COUNSELLING

*A. E. H. Emery*

D URING the last few decades there has been a gradual decline in the incidence of infectious diseases and nutritional deficiencies. Their place is being taken by disorders which are largely, if not entirely, genetic in causation, and such disorders are therefore becoming increasingly important in medical practice.

Genetic counselling is concerned with advising parents on the risks of recurrence of hereditary disorders and therefore indirectly with the prevention of these disorders. The purpose of genetic counselling is fourfold. Firstly, to explain as simply as possible the nature of the disorder and what is meant by saying that it is 'genetic'. Secondly, to dispel feelings of guilt which parents often have who have borne a child with such a disorder. Thirdly, to explain the risks of recurrence and finally, give appropriate advice when this is requested. The purpose of this brief review is to present some of the basic principles underlying genetic counselling.

## UNIFACTORIAL INHERITANCE

It is useful to consider human disease as falling on a spectrum. At one extreme there are those conditions which are almost entirely genetic in causation such as haemophilia where the environment seems to play no direct part in aetiology. At the other end of the spectrum there are the nutritional deficiencies and infectious diseases which are almost entirely due to environmental factors. Between the two extremes there are many fairly common conditions, such as diabetes mellitus and certain congenital malformations (pyloric stenosis, dislocation of the hip club foot) in which both genetic and environmental factors are involved.

Those disorders which are entirely genetic in causation are either chromosomal abnormalities or are due to single gene mutations (*unifactorial*). The latter are rare, the mode of inheritance is simple (dominant, recessive or X-linked) and the chances of recurrence are high (greater than 1 in 10).

Those disorders which are partly genetic in causation are due to many genes and the effects of environment (*multifactorial*). These disorders are common, the mode of inheritance is complex and the chances of recurrence are usually low (less than 1 in 10).

For many characteristics or traits each individual possesses two genes. If an individual possesses two genes which are the same he is said to be *homozygous* for that particular trait. If the two genes are different, he is *heterozygous*. A gene which is manifest in the heterozygote is *dominant*, whereas a gene which is manifest only in the homozygote is *recessive*. The terms *dominant* and *recessive* do not refer to characteristics of the genes themselves but only to their manifestations (traits). It is therefore incorrect for example, to refer to a 'dominant gene' but rather to a 'dominant trait' or 'dominant disorder'.

A trait which is determined by a gene on an *autosome* is said to be inherited as an autosomal trait and may be dominant or recessive. A trait which is determined by a gene on one of the sex chromosomes is said to be sex-

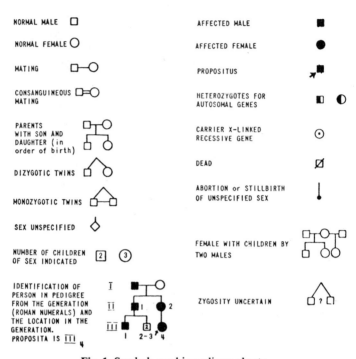

**Fig. 1.** Symbols used in pedigree charts.

linked and may also be either dominant or recessive.

It is a rule in genetics that only one of a pair of genes (=*alleles*) is transmitted to any particular offspring and it is purely a matter of chance which allele happens to be transmitted at any one time.

### Drawing the family tree

Before giving genetic counselling it is essential to draw up a family tree which, as a minimum, should include information on the health of all first-degree relatives, *i.e.* parents, brothers and sisters (sibs) and children of the person seeking such advice.

Drawing up the family tree begins with the affected person first found to have the trait in a family. This is the *index case* or *proband* and is indicated by an arrow. In any generation, sibs are arranged in decreasing age from

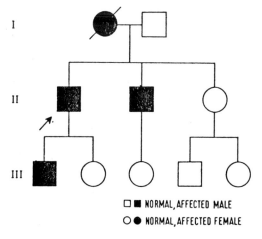

□ ■ NORMAL, AFFECTED MALE
○ ● NORMAL, AFFECTED FEMALE

**Fig. 2.** Pedigree pattern of an autosomal dominant trait.

left to right. The symbols used in pedigree charts are given in Figure 1.

### Autosomal dominant inheritance

A person heterozygous for an autosomal dominant trait possesses the abnormal (mutant) gene which causes the disorder as well as its normal allels.

If the disorder is not severe then it may be possible to trace it back through several generations (Fig. 2) but if the condition is severe, affected individuals may not survive to have children and so transmit the disease to subsequent generations. In such cases the affected individual is 'sporadic' being the only affected person in the family, and usually the result of a new mutation. For example, about 80 per cent of patients with achondroplasia are the result of new mutations.

Autosomal dominant traits affect both males and females and often show great variation in severity (=*expressivity*). **For** example in osteogenesis imperfecta (brittle bones) the only manifestation of the disease may be blue sclerae but other individuals even in the same family can be very severely affected with multiple fractures present at birth.

47

Sometimes the gene may not express itself at all in which case it is said to be *non-penetrant*. This phenomenon explains apparent 'skipped' generations in certain pedigrees (*e.g.* tuberose sclerosis). However, in many such cases careful examination often shows that the 'skipped individual' has definite although mild manifestations, and is sometimes referred to as *forme fruste*. Careful clinical examination of both apparently healthy parents of a child with an autosomal dominant disorder is therefore essential before the possibility of a new mutation can be considered.

If an affected individual marries a normal person on *average* half their children will be affected. The reason is that each gamete of an affected person carries either the normal gene or the gene for the trait. If the gene for the normal (recessive) trait is represented as *a*, and the gene for the abnormal (dominant) trait as *A*, then the various gametic combinations are:

|  | | Affected parent (Aa) ↓ gametes | |
|  | | A | a |
| --- | --- | --- | --- |
| Normal parent → gametes (aa) | a | Aa affected | aa normal |
|  | a | Aa affected | aa normal |

The chance that any child may be affected is therefore 50 per cent or 1 in 2.

Some autosomal genes are expressed more frequently in one sex than the other. This is referred to as *sex-influenced* inheritance, or sex-limited inheritance in the extreme case in which only one sex is affected. A possible example of a sex-influenced autosomal dominant trait is haemochromatosis which is much commoner in males than females who often do not develop symptoms until after the menopause.

In the testicular feminization syndrome only males are affected and they are infertile, the condition being transmitted by healthy females. It has so far not been possible to decide whether this is an autosomal dominant trait with male limitation or a sex-linked recessive trait.

## Autosomal recessive inheritance

Autosomal recessive traits affect both sexes and since only homozygotes are affected the parents, who must be heterozygotes, are perfectly healthy. Therefore unlike an autosomal dominant trait it is not possible to trace the disease through several generations. All the affected individuals in a family are usually in one sibship, that is they are brothers and sisters (Fig. 3).

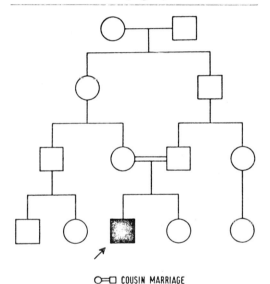

○═□ COUSIN MARRIAGE

**Fig. 3.** Pedigree pattern of an autosomal recessive trait.

The parents of a child with a rare recessive disorder are often related, the reason being that cousins are more likely to carry the same gene having inherited it from a common ancestor. The rarer a disorder the more likely it is that the parents will be related, but if in a particular family the parents are not related this does not of course preclude the condition from being a recessive trait. On *average* one in four of the offspring of two heterozygotes are affected. If the gene for the normal (dominant) trait is represented as $A$, and the gene for the abnormal (recessive) trait is $a$, then the various gametic combinations are:

Normal heterozygous parent (Aa)
↓
gametes

|  | A | a |
|---|---|---|
| A | AA<br>normal | Aa<br>unaffected<br>heterozygote |
| a | Aa<br>unaffected<br>heterozygote | aa<br>affected |

Normal heterozygous parent→gametes (Aa)

Nowadays since families tend to be small it often happens that autosomal recessive conditions are sporadic with only one affected person in the family.

As a general rule autosomal recessive traits are often due to an enzyme defect whereas autosomal dominant traits are usually due to an abnormality of a non-enzymatic protein (*e.g.* collagen).

### X-linked recessive inheritance

Apart from hairy ears, no Mendelizing genes are known to be carried on the Y chromosome, therefore, sex-linkage is essentially synonymous with X-linkage.

An X-linked recessive trait is one which is due to a mutant gene on the X chromosome. Hemizygous males (with the mutant gene on

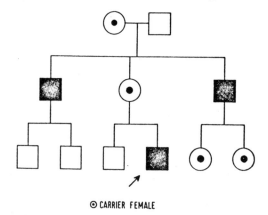

⊙ CARRIER FEMALE

Fig. 4. Pedigree pattern of an X-linked recessive trait in which affected males reproduce.

their single X chromosome) are affected but heterozygous females (=*carriers*) are usually perfectly healthy. Diseases inherited in this manner (Fig. 4) are transmitted by healthy female carriers and by affected males if the disorder is not severe or is treatable. Haemophilia is an X-linked recessive disorder where improvements in medical treatment and surgical techniques have led to affected males often surviving into adult life. If an affected male marries a normal female and if the haemopilia gene is represented as Xh and the normal gene as X, then the various gametic combinations can be represented as:

Affected male (XhY)
↓
gametes

|  |  | Xh | Y |
|---|---|---|---|
| Normal female→gametes (XX) | X | XXh carrier daughter | XY normal son |
| | X | XXh carrier daughter | XY normal son |

Thus, all the daughters of an affected male will be carriers and all his sons will be normal. In severe X-linked disorders, such as Duchenne muscular dystrophy, affected males do not survive to have children and the disorder is entirely transmitted by female carriers (Fig. 5). In the case of a woman who is a carrier of Duchenne muscular dystrophy (XdX) and marries a normal male then half her sons will be affected and half her daughters will be carriers:

Carrier female (XdX)
↓
gametes

|  |  | Xd | X |
|---|---|---|---|
| Normal male→gametes (XY) | X | XXd carrier daughter | XX normal daughter |
| | Y | XdY affected son | YX normal son |

51

Quite often in serious X-linked conditions there is only one affected boy in a family. Such a sporadic case may be the result of a new mutation in the X-chromosome which the boy inherited from his mother. There is also the possibility however, that the mother might be a carrier, the mutant gene by chance not having been transmitted to any of her male relatives but inherited only through the female line perhaps for several generations.

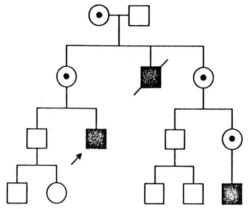

**Fig. 5.** Pedigree pattern of a severe X-linked recessive trait in which affected males do not survive to have children.

**GENETIC HETEROGENEITY**

It is now well recognised that clinically similar or seemingly identical disorders may be inherited differently which indicates that such disorders must be different disease entities. The recognition of the existence of different genetic disorders within one particular disease (=*genetic heterogeneity*) is essential for reliable genetic counselling.

Different genes which produce clinically identical disorders are sometimes referred to as *mimic* genes. Examples include hereditary spastic paraplegia, peroneal muscular atrophy and retinitis pigmentosa each of which in any particular family may be inherited as an autosomal dominant trait, or as an autosomal recessive trait or as an X-linked recessive trait. In such circumstances the recessive form is usually more severe than the dominant form and the X-linked form tends to be

52

intermediate in severity. This is sometimes referred to as Allen's law.

There are other disorders which are inherited in an identical manner but can be subdivided on the basis of either the clinical findings as in the severe Duchenne and benign Becker types of X-linked muscular dystrophy or biochemical tests as in the A (classical) and B (Christmas disease) types of X-linked haemophilia and the various autosomal recessive forms of nonspherocytic haemolytic anaemia (*e.g.* pyruvate kinase deficiency, triosephosphate isomerase deficiency, glutathione deficiency and glutathione reductase deficiency).

Some other disorders which are genetically heterogeneous include the mucopolysaccharidoses (McKusick *et al.*, 1965), the muscular dystrophies (Emery & Walton, 1967) and the chondrodystrophies (McKusick, 1968).

## MULTIFACTORIAL INHERITANCE

There are many fairly common conditions in which there is a definite familial tendency, the proportion of affected relatives being greater than in the general population. However the proportion of affected relatives is often of the order of 5 per cent and, therefore, much less than would be expected for a unifactorial trait. It has sometimes been suggested that the low familial incidence in such conditions might be because the responsible gene was 'incompletely penetrant'. This explanation however, is rather unsatisfactory for several reasons and it is much more likely that such conditions are caused by many genes and the effects of environment, so-called *multifactorial* inheritance.

In multifactorial inheritance it is assumed that there is some hypothetical underlying graded attribute which is related to the causation of the disease. This is referred to as the individual's *liability*, which includes not only his genetic predisposition but also the environmental circumstances which render him more or less likely to develop the disease. It is assumed in multifactorial inheritance

53

that the curve of liability has a normal distribution in both the general population and in relatives (Fig. 6) but the curve for relatives is shifted to the right. The points on the curves above which all individuals are

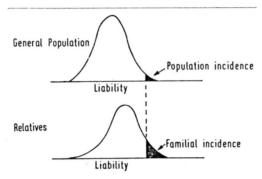

Fig. 6. Hypothetical curve of liability in the general population and in relatives for a hereditary disorder in which the genetic predisposition is multifactorial.

affected is the threshold. In the general population the proportion above the threshold is the population incidence and among relatives the proportion above the threshold is the familial incidence (Fig. 6). This model has been applied to measurable characters (such as stature and intelligence) and also to explain the familial incidence of such conditions as diabetes mellitus, congenital pyloric stenosis, hare lip with and without cleft palate, anencephaly and spina bifida, club foot and congenital dislocation of the hip (Carter, 1965, 1969). It may also be the explanation for ischaemic heart disease, ankylosing spondylitis, peptic ulcer, strabismus and the commoner forms of congenital heart disease.

In conditions in which the inheritance is believed to be multifactorial there are several consequences of such a model. The incidence will be greatest among the relatives of more severely affected individuals because presumably they are more extreme deviants along the curve of liability. Thus in hare lip with or without cleft palate the proportion of affected relatives (sibs and children) is roughly 6 per cent (1 in 16) when the index patient has doubled hare lip and cleft palate, but only 2.5 per cent (1 in 40) if he only has a single hare lip (Carter, 1965). By similar reasoning it would also be expected that the incidence among sibs born subsequent to the index case would be greater the more affected relatives there were in the family. In spina bifida for example, after the birth of a single affected child the incidence among subsequent sibs is approximately 4 per cent, but 10 per cent after the birth of 2 affected children and evidence suggests the risk is higher still if another close relative is also affected. This is quite different from the situation in unifactorial traits where the risk in subsequent sibs remains constant irrespective of the number of affected individuals in the family already (*e.g.* 1 in 4 for an autosomal recessive trait).

Finally in multifactorial inheritance it follows that when there is a sex difference in the population incidence, the relatives of the less frequently affected sex will be more often affected. The explanation in this case is probably that the curve of liability has the same distribution in both sexes but that of the less frequently affected sex is shifted to the left so that they are more extreme when they are affected. Thus, in pyloric stenosis which is 5 times commoner in boys than girls, the proportions of affected relatives of male index patients are 5.5 per cent for sons and 2.4 per cent for daughters, but 19.4 per cent for sons and 7.3 per cent for daughters when the index patient is a female (Carter, 1969).

### DETERMINATION OF RECURRENCE RISKS

Estimation of the risks of recurrence in the individual case depends upon a precise diagnosis and an established aetiology. Before giving genetic counselling a careful clinical examination and investigation of the affected individual, is therefore, essential. In order to arrive at the correct diagnosis, it may be necessary to refer to death certificates and autopsy and biopsy reports and it may also be necessary to examine the parents in certain situations. Without this information it may not be possible to give reliable genetic counselling.

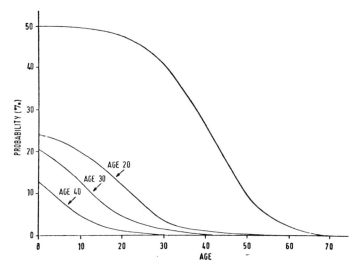

**Fig. 7.** Probability that a healthy man and his son (born when his father was aged 20, 30 or 40 years) may have inherited Huntington's chorea from a grandparent.

In establishing the aetiology a pedigree must be drawn up which includes information on the health of at least all first-degree relatives, consanguinity, abortions, maternal exposure to radiation, drugs and infections during pregnancy and details of any birth trauma. Finally the possibility of genetic heterogeneity must always be remembered. The literature should be searched for information on this point and also on the relative frequencies of the various modes of inheritance. The subject is dealt with in greater detail elsewhere (Reed, 1963; Motulsky & Hecht, 1964; Townes, 1966; Emery, 1968).

### Calculation of probabilities

In calculating the probability of an individual being affected with an hereditary disorder we are usually only concerned with the so-called *prior* probability; that is the probability based on information about the individual's antecedents. If the condition is either an autosomal trait with variable age of onset or an X-linked recessive trait, then it is necessary to take into account the so-called *conditional probability*. This is the probability that a person may be affected (or be a carrier) depending on their age or the results of

56

various biochemical tests. From the prior and conditional probabilities it is possible to calculate the *joint* probability which is the product of the prior and conditional probabilities. Finally, the *relative* probability is calculated, which is the joint probability of being affected (or of being a carrier) divided by this probability plus the joint probability of *not* being affected. Thus, a man of 50 who is healthy but whose father died of Huntington's chorea (an autosomal dominant trait, with age of onset between 25 and 55 years, and where 80 per cent of cases develop symptoms before age 50 years), the chance (relative probability) that he may have inherited the disorder but has so far remained healthy is calculated as follows:

| Probability | Inherited the disorder | Not inherited the disorder |
|---|---|---|
| Prior | 1/2 | 1/2 |
| Conditional | 1/5 * | 1 |
| Joint | 1/10 | 1/2 |
| Relative | $\dfrac{1/10}{1/10 + 1/2} = 1/6$ | |

(*the probability that by age 50 years he would not have manifested the disease even if he had inherited the disorder)

The probability that this man's son may have inherited the gene is therefore 1 in 12. Of course as each year goes by and the father remains healthy so his risks of having inherited Huntington's chorea decrease (Fig. 7).

## Recurrence risks in rare genetic disorders

When the precise diagnosis is known and the mode of inheritance clearly established (Table I) genetic counselling is usually straightforward and is based on Mendelian ratios which have already been discussed. It should be remembered however, that in the case of autosomal recessive conditions a parent, whether homozygous or heterozygous, is unlikely to have affected children unless he or she happens to marry someone who carries the same mutant gene and this is unlikely if the condition is rare.

**Table I.** Modes of inheritance of some genetic (unifactorial) disorders. To date none of these particular disorders appears to exhibit genetic heterogeneity.

| Autosomal dominant | Autosomal recessive | X-linked recessive |
|---|---|---|
| Achondroplasia | Adrenal hyperplasia | Aldrich syndrome |
| Dubin-Johnson's disease | Albinism | Choroideremia |
| Ehlers-Danlos syndrome | Alkaptonuria | Deutan & Protan colour blindness |
| Facio-scapulo-humeral muscular dystrophy | Amaurotic idiocy | Duchenne muscular dystrophy |
| Haemoglobin variants | Ataxia telangiectasia | G-6-PD deficiency |
| Holt-Oram syndrome | Crigler-Najjar syndrome | Fabry's disease |
| Huntington's chorea | Fibrocystic disease | Granulomatous dis. of childhood |
| Marfan's syndrome | Dysautonomia | Haemophilia A & B |
| Myotonia congenita | Friedreich's ataxia | Hunter's syndrome |
| Neurofibromatosis | Galactosaemia | Nephrogenic diabetes insipidus |
| Periodic Paralyses | Hartnup's disease | Ocular albinism |
| Polyposis coli | Homocystinuria | Oculo-cerebro-renal syndrome |
| Porphyria variegata | Hurler's syndrome | Retinoschisis |
| Tuberose sclerosis | Laurence-Moon-Biedl syndrome | |
| Waardenburg's syndrome | Limb girdle muscular dystrophy | |
| | Maple syrup urine disease | |
| | Niemann-Pick's disease | |
| | Oroticaciduria | |
| | Phenylketonuria | |
| | Pendred's syndrome | |
| | Pseudoxanthoma | |
| | Refsum's syndrome | |
| | Werdnig-Hoffman's disease | |
| | Wilson's disease | |

**Table II.** Empiric risks (%) for some common disorders.

| Disorder | Incidence | Sex ratio M:F | Normal parents having a second affected child | Affected parent having an affected child | Affected parent having a second affected child |
|---|---|---|---|---|---|
| Anencephaly | 0.20 | 1:2 | 2 | — | — |
| Cleft palate only | 0.04 | 2:3 | 2 | 7 | 15 |
| Cleft lip ± cleft palate | 0.10 | 3:2 | 4 | 4 | 12 |
| Club foot | 0.10 | 2:1 | 3 | 3 | 10 |
| Cong. heart disease (all types) | 0.60 | — | 1-4 | 1-4 | — |
| Diabetes mellitus (early onset) | 0.10 | 1:1 | 3 | 3 | 10 |
| Dislocation of hip | 0.07 | 1:6 | 4 | 4 | 10 |
| Epilepsy ('idiopathic') | 0.50 | 1:1 | 5 | 5 | 10 |
| Hirschsprung's disease | 0.02 | 4:1 | | — | |
|   male index | | | 2 | | |
|   female index | | | 8 | | |
| Manic-depressive psychoses | 0.40 | 2:3 | 10-15 | 10-15 | — |
| Mental retardation ('idiopathic') | 0.30 -0.50 | 1:1 | 3-5 | | — |
| Pyloric stenosis | 0.30 | 5:1 | | | |
|   male index | | | 2 | 4 | 13 |
|   female index | | | 10 | 17 | 38 |
| Schizophrenia | 1.00 | 1:1 | 8 | 12 | — |
| Scoliosis (idiopathic, adolescent) | 0.22 | 1:6 | 7 | 5 | — |
| Spina bifida | 0.30 | 2:3 | 4 | — | — |

### Recurrence risks in common genetic disorders

In fairly common conditions in which genetic factors appear to play a part but where there is no simple mode of inheritance, the risks of recurrence are based on the observed frequencies of the conditions among relatives of affected individuals, so-called *empiric risks* (Table II). Many of these conditions are probably heterogeneous and include disorders of various causation. Empiric risk figures are therefore rather unsatisfactory as they merely represent an 'average figure' for any one condition and there is always the possibility that the disorder in a particular family might be unifactorial with a high risk (*e.g.* 1 in 4) of recurrence. Further, such risk figures should not be applied in the individual case without some qualification because, as we have seen, they depend to some extent upon the sex and severity of the condition in the index patient and the number of affected persons in the family.

If a genetic aetiology for a particular condition has not been established and yet the family history clearly suggests a particular mode of inheritance then genetic counselling should be based on the family history since this condition may represent a unique situation (a 'private' genotype). Townes (1966), for example, has reported a family in which congenital malrotation of the colon recurred in several sibs yet no familial cases had been reported in the literature. Again there are other conditions which may present as a *phenocopy* (resembles a genetically determined condition but is not inherited). For example, bilateral retinoblastoma is often familial and inherited as an autosomal dominant trait but many unilateral cases are probably phenocopies and an affected person has a low risk of having an affected child.

### Recurrence risks in chromosome abnormalities

In general trisomy-21 (Down's syndrome) trisomy-D, trisomy-E, anti-mongolism, cri du chat syndrome, Klinefelter's syndrome and Turner's syndrome are usually the result of

**Table III.** Risks of recurrence of Down's syndrome due to various chromosome abnormalities. C = carrier; N = normal.

| Patient | Karyotypes | | Chance of recurrence |
|---|---|---|---|
| | Father | Mother | |
| Translocation: | | | |
| 13-15/21-22 | N | C | 10-20% |
| | C | N | 5% |
| 21/22 | N | C | 10-20% |
| | C | N | 5% |
| 21/21 | C | N | 100% |
| | N | C | 100% |
| Trisomy-21 | N | N | <5% |
| Translocation or mosaic | | | Small |

61

errors in meiosis during gametogenesis and the chances of recurrence are small. If, however, one of the parents happens to be a mosaic- or carries a balanced translocation the situation is different. When one of the parents is a mosaic it is very difficult to give reliable genetic counselling because it is impossible to estimate what proportion of the parental gonadal tissue is normal. If one of the parents carries a translocation, genetic counselling depends upon the cytogenetic findings which, in the case of Down's syndrome, are summarised in Table III. Over 95 per cent of cases of Down's syndrome have trisomy-21 and the chances of recurrence depend on the mother's age being about 1 in 800 at age 25 years rising to about 1 in 20 at age 45 years.

### Genetic counselling and the sporadic case

A common problem is when healthy parents have a child with a particular disorder or abnormality and there is no family history of anyone on either side of the family having been similarly affected. There are several possible explanations for this. Firstly, it might be a phenocopy perhaps due to something to which the mother was exposed during pregnancy (*e.g.* there is about a 1 in 5 chance that a mother infected with rubella in early pregnancy may have a child with one or more major defects such as microcephaly, cataracts, congenital heart disease and deafness). Secondly, it may be due to a chromosome abnormality, but apart from Down's syndrome, the other syndromes associated with *specific* chromosome abnormalities (*e.g.* trisomy-D, trisomy-E, cri du chat syndrome) are very rare and the chances of recurrence are small.

A third possibility is that it may represent an autosomal dominant new mutation in which case there is little chance of recurrence in subsequent children. This is a distinct possibility if the condition is known to be always inherited as an autosomal dominant trait and is always fully penetrant and if both parents have been carefully examined and

**Table IV.** Carrier detection in X-linked disorders.

These have been arbitrarily divided into two groups:
(1) the proportion detectable exceeds 50 per cent.
(2) the proportion detectable is uncertain because so far too few carriers have been studied.

| Disorder | Abnormality |
|---|---|
| **Group 1** Haemophilia **A** | factor VIII reduced |
| Haemophilia **B** | factor IX reduced |
| G-6-PD deficiency | erythrocyte G-6-PD reduced |
| Congenital agammaglobulinaemia | *in vitro* immunoglobulin synthesis by lymphocytes reduced |
| Lesch-Nyhan syndrome | hypoxanthine-guanine phosphoribosyl transferase in skin fibroblasts reduced. Two populations of cells. |
| Hunter's syndrome | granules in skin fibroblasts |
| Choroideremia | patchy pigmentation of retina |
| Ocular albinism | patchy depigmentation of retina and iris |
| Retinitis pigmentosa | tapetoretinal reflex |
| Vit. D resistant rickets (hypophosphataemia) | serum phosphorus reduced |
| Duchenne muscular dystrophy | serum creatine kinase raised |
| Becker muscular dystrophy | serum creatine kinase raised |
| Diabetes insipidus (nephrogenic) | urine concentration diminished |
| **Group 2** Fabry's disease (angiokeratoma) | urinary glycolipids (ceramide hexosides) increased |
| Keratosis follicularis (Siemens) | Skin and corneal abnormalities |
| Anhidrotic ectodermal dysplasia | patchy sweating |
| Lowe syndrome (Oculo-cerebro-renal) | lenticular opacities by slit lamp |
| Aldrich syndrome | platelet count reduced |
| Pyridoxine-responsive anaemia (Rundles-Falls) | minor erythrocyte abnormalities |
| Congenital dysphagocytosis (fatal granulomatous disease of childhood) | phagocytosis histochemical test abnormal |

63

been found to be perfectly healthy.

Fourthly, it might be an autosomal recessive disorder. Evidence in favour of this would be if the parents were cousins or if by an appropriate biochemical or other test *both* parents could be shown to be heterozygotes.

Finally, it could be an X-linked recessive disorder. It is important to recognise this possibility because an unaffected sister might then be a carrier. Clinical evidence might suggest the mode of inheritance (*e.g.* clouding of the cornea is present in autosomal recessive Hurler's syndrome but not in the clinically similar X-linked recessive Hunter's syndrome) or one form may be much more likely than another (the X-linked type of Duchenne muscular dystrophy is at least ten times more frequent than the autosomal recessive form of this disease). It might also be possible to demonstrate an appropriate biochemical or other abnormality in the mother but not in the father which would suggest that the disorder was X-linked (Table IV).

**Genetic counselling in X-linked disorders where a suspected carrier has a normal test result**

Tests are now available by means of which it is possible to detect symptomless female carriers of many X-linked disorders (Table IV). Unfortunately in some of these conditions the proportion of carriers who can be detected is not 100 per cent. The problem of counselling a suspected carrier who has a normal test result can be resolved by using the method of calculating probabilities as discussed on page 345.

In an X-linked lethal disorder, such as Duchenne muscular dystrophy, the prior probability of a woman being a carrier as the result of a new mutation in either her father's sperm or her mother's ovum is $2\mu$ where $\mu$ is the mutation rate and is approximately equal to $5 \times 10^{-5}$ in Duchenne muscular dystrophy. The probability that she may have inherited the mutant gene from her mother is also $2\mu$ and therefore the total prior probability of her being a carrier is $4\mu$. In this laboratory it has been found that approximately two-thirds of known carriers have serum levels of creatine kinase greater than the normal 95 percentile. If a suspected carrier has two sons one of whom is affected, and if her serum level of creatine kinase is less than the normal 95 percentile then:

| Probability | | Carrier | Not a carrier |
|---|---|---|---|
| Prior | | $4\mu$ | $1-4\mu \simeq 1$ |
| *conditional: | genetic | $\left(\frac{1}{2}\right)^2$ | $\mu$ (new mutation) |
| | biochemical | $\frac{1}{3}$ | $\frac{19}{20}$ |
| Joint | | $\frac{\mu}{3}$ | $\frac{19}{20}\mu$ |
| relative | | 0.26 | 0.74 |

* (the probability of having one affected and one normal son and a "normal" serum level of creatine kinase assuming the woman is or is not a carrier)

In this way it is possible to derive a general formula for calculating the probability of a woman being a carrier of a lethal X-linked disorder. If $h_c$ and $h_m$, based on the results of biochemical and other tests, refer respectively to the relative chances of normal homozygosity to heterozygosity in the suspected carrier and her mother such that if there is no such information $h = 1$, and
if $q =$ number of normal brothers
$r =$ number of normal sons
$s = 1$ where a son is affected and
      0 if a brother is affected
$t = 0$ where a son is affected and
      1 if a brother is affected
then the probability (P) of a woman being a carrier of a lethal X-linked disorder *when there is only one affected person in the family* (a son or brother):

$$= \frac{1 + sa}{1 + sa + ab + tb}$$

where $a = h_m 2^q$ and $b = h_c 2^r$. The relative chances of normal homozygosity to heterozygosity (h) can be estimated from knowing the proportions of normal healthy women and known carriers with a test result the same as the suspected carrier. For example in the case of carriers of Duchenne muscular

Table V. Relative probabilities of normal homozygosity to heterozygosity (Y1/Y2 = h) for various serum levels of creatine kinase.

| Serum CK | Controls | | Carriers | | h (Y1/Y2) |
|---|---|---|---|---|---|
| | No. | %(Y1) | No. | %(Y2) | |
| 0-10 | 1 | 1 | 0 | 0.0 | *46.24 |
| 11-20 | 18 | 18 | 0 | 0.0 | *18.20 |
| 21-30 | 51 | 51 | 3 | 8.6 | 5.93 |
| 31-40 | 16 | 16 | 2 | 5.7 | 2.81 |
| 41-50 | 8 | 8 | 3 | 8.6 | 0.93 |
| 51-60 | 5 | 5 | 4 | 11.4 | 0.44 |
| 61-70 | 1 | 1 | 2 | 5.7 | 0.18 |
| >70 | 0 | 0 | 21 | 60.0 | — |
| Total | 100 | 100 | 35 | 100.0 | |

(*values obtained by extrapolation)

66

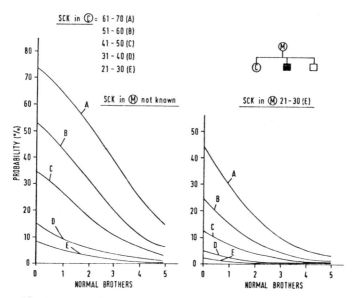

**Fig. 8.** Probability of a woman being a carrier of Duchenne muscular dystrophy who has an affected brother and several normal brothers.

dystrophy, values of h have been obtained (Table V) from serum levels of creatine kinase determined according to the method of Rosalki (1967). Results obtained by substituting various values of h from Table V in the above formula are illustrated in Figure 8. The likelihood of a woman being a carrier of Duchenne muscular dystrophy who has an affected brother, is less the lower her serum level of creatine kinase and the more normal brothers she has since this makes it more likely that her affected brother is the result of a new mutation. If her mother also has a low serum level of creatine kinase the probability of being a carrier may work out to be within acceptable limits (Fig. 8). This example illustrates very well that in such conditions as Duchenne muscular dystrophy in order to give reliable genetic counselling when there is only one affected male in the family it is essential to test not only the suspected carrier but also her mother. Of course if an appropriate test indicates that the woman is a definite carrier

**Table VI.** Possibilities open to parents who have had a child with a particular hereditary disorder, or are themselves affected (e.g. osteogenesis imperfecta) or carry a particular chromosome translocation (Down's syndrome).
*Selective abortion possible

| Example | risk (%) | contraception | sterilization | abortion |
|---|---|---|---|---|
| Cleft palate alone | 2 | — | — | — |
| Spina bifida (1 affected child) | 4 | ? | — | ? |
| Spina bifida (2 affected children) | 10 | ++ | ? | ++* |
| Galactosaemia | 25 | ++ | ++ | ++* |
| Duchenne muscular dystrophy | 50 (sons) | + | ++ | +* |
|  | 50 (daughters) | + |  |  |
| Osteogenesis imperfecta | 50 | + | + | + |
| Down's syndrome |  |  |  |  |
| 13/15 translocation | 5-20 | ++ | ++ | ++* |
| 21/21 translocation | 100 | ++ | ++ | ++ |

or if there is more than one affected male in the family, then genetic counselling can be based on first principles and this more eleborate approach is not necessary.

**Genetic advice**

Factors which influence the parents' decision as to whether or not they will accept the risk of having an affected child include the severity of the abnormality, whether there is an effective treatment, the actual risk, their religious attitudes and socio-economic status and education. The genetic counsellor usually does not try to influence the parents' decision. However, in one study (Carter, 1967) about a quarter of high risk families planned further children despite the risks involved. This suggests that perhaps the genetic counsellor, at least in the case of serious genetic disorders with a high risk of recurrence, should do more than merely explain the risks. Perhaps he should suggest in such cases that family limitation would be advisable.

Contraception is not the only course of action open to the parents (Table VI). Other possibilities include sterilization, artificial insemination by donor (if the father is affected) and, with the liberalisation of the Abortion Law, if there is a 'substantial risk' of a serious abnormality then termination is possible should the mother become pregnant. Recently *selective* abortion has also become a possibility whereby a pregnancy need only be terminated when it is *known* that the foetus is abnormal. This is possible by removing a small amount (2-5 ml.) of amniotic fluid by transabdominal amniocentesis around the 12th to 20th weeks of gestation and carrying out sex-chromatin, chromosome and biochemical studies on the contained cells (Emery *et al.*, 1969). A known carrier of an X-linked disorder which cannot yet be diagnosed *in utero* might choose selective abortion of a male foetus rather than the only other alternative of totally restricting her family. In certain disorders, such as galactosaemia, antenatal diagnosis is now possible and foetuses known to be affected may be selectively aborted. Parents who have already had an affected child can thus be guaranteed a healthy child in a subsequent pregnancy.

## Genetic register

We have accumulated evidence which clearly suggests that there is a significant number of persons in the population who are at high risk of having a child with a serious hereditary disorder but are unaware of this. In the past the ascertainment of such individuals has often been a matter of chance depending largely on the awareness of their medical attendant. There is an important need therefore to set up genetic registers in which families at high risk are recorded so that individuals in these families can be followed up and given appropriate counselling. The setting up and usefulness of genetic registers has been discussed in detail recently by Smith (1969).

## CONCLUSIONS

In giving genetic counselling it is not sufficient merely to quote risk figures but, as far as this is possible, the nature and cause of the disease should be explained to the parents. Feelings of guilt and misconceptions about aetiology should be removed. Other problems may also have to be discussed including child adoption, abortion, sterilization and perhaps even artificial insemination by donor. Since the consequences of genetic counselling can be profound and far reaching such advice should never be given lightly. It involves not only familiarity with the medical and genetic aspects of hereditary disease but also an awareness of the personal problems which are often involved. Genetic counselling is essentially one aspect of clinical medicine.

REFERENCES

Carter, C. O. (1965). The inheritance of common congenital malformations. *Progress in Medical Genetics*, **4**, 59-84

Carter, C. O. (1967). Comments on genetic counselling. In *Proceedings of the IIIrd International Congress of Human Genetics*, p. 97. Baltimore: Johns Hopkins Press

Carter, C. O. (1969). Genetics of common disorders. *British Medical Bulletin,* **25,** 52

Emery, A. E. H. (1968). *Elements of Medical Genetics* Edinburgh: Livingstone

Emery, A. E. H., Nelson, M. M., Gordon, G., Burt, D. (1969). Antenatal Diagnosis. *Scottish Medical Journal,* **14,** 277

Emery, A. E. H., Walton, J. N. (1967). The genetics of muscular dystrophy. *Progress in Medical Genetics,* **5,** 116

McKusick, V. A. (1968). *Mendelian Inheritance in Man,* 2nd edition. London: Heinemann

McKusick, V. A., Kaplan, D., Wise, D., Hanley, W. B., Suddarth, S. B., Sevick, M. E., Maumanee, A. E. (1965). The genetic mucopolysaccharidoses. *Medicine,* **44,** 445

Motulsky, A. G., Hecht, F. (1964). Genetic prognosis and counselling. *American Journal of Obstetrics and Gynecology,* **90,** 1227

Reed, S. C. (1963). *Counselling in Medical Genetics.* Philadelphia: Saunders

Rosalki, S. B. (1967). An improved procedure for serum creatine phosphokinase determination. *Journal of Laboratory and Clinical Medicine,* **69,** 696

Smith, C. (1969). Ascertaining those at risk in the prevention and treatment of genetic disease. In *Modern Trends in Human Genetics.* London: Butterworth. (in press)

Townes, P. L. (1966). Genetic counselling. *Pediatric Clinics North America,* **13,** 337

# Progress in

# the Delivery of Health Care

Kathleen Taylor, MSW
Robert E. Merrill, MD

Genetic counseling should be a regular and effective part of any health care program. This survey of 21 families encompassing 24 boys with typical Duchenne X-linked progressive muscular dystrophy demonstrates that genetic information has not been effectively provided to this group. How social workers and others could contribute to an effective model teaching program is emphasized. The ultimate goal is the general implementation of established principles leading to effective preventive pediatrics.

It is appropriate that physicians and others concerned with the delivery of health care are concerned with all aspects of disease prevention. We recognize that, as a preventive measure, genetic counseling can be a complex process, requiring the talents of the geneticist. Yet for many severely crippling diseases, based on current knowledge, the patterns of inheritance are well enough established to allow the practicing physician to discuss probabilities with confidence. Provided diagnosis is accurate, hemophilia, X-linked progressive muscular dystro-

phy, and mucoviscidosis represent challenges of this sort. It should be possible for the physician to share enough basic information with young parents of individuals with these and other similar diseases to allow them to make rational decisions regarding whether to have more children or not. The application of well established facts could be an effective measure in the prevention of needless suffering in a family, thus making unnecessary the medical care required to alleviate that distress.

Ideally, all practicing physicians regularly invoke this sort of counseling. We have no accurate information on the point, but the common failure of pediatric house officers in training to consider such aspects made us wonder how many opportunities for this kind of preventive pediatrics are recognized by the pediatric practitioners.

These doubts led us to wonder about our own performance in a clinic designed to provide longitudinal care for children with X-linked progressive muscular dystrophy. In theory, demonstration of excellent counseling by us would lead to similar practice by the house officers both while in training and later.

This paper summarizes our lack of success in providing useful information to families containing boys with progressive muscular dystrophy and contains a proposal for a method of correction.

We believe that the clinic staff has a clear obligation to provide information to the patients and families regarding the nature and transmission of disease. Whether decisions for families should be made by the staff is questionable, but where inheritance patterns are reasonably clear, the staff should provide understandable information to the families with the hope that they may make rational decisions. Family planning decisions are especially important at this time when no effective therapy for progressive muscular dystrophy exists and because of the impact of this disease on the affected family.

That our point of view is neither unprecedented nor unrealistic is supported by several authors. Both physicians [1] and social workers [2,3] have advocated action in this area and have outlined the challenges and opportunities. That genetic information could have been useful has been well documented.[4]

## Patient Material

The roster of all patients regularly attending a muscular dystrophy clinic was searched. The patients and their families were selected for study if the index patient was a male subject, if no female subjects in the family were affected with the disease, and if the disease appeared to be gradually progressive at a pace (with one exception) which suggested that complete immobility and death would occur in the late second or early third decade of life. A variety of procedures had been used to make the diagnosis, including electromyography, muscle biopsy, and enzyme studies. When done, the test supported the diagnosis of progressive muscular dystrophy of the X-linked Duchenne type. It is emphasized that selection for study was primarily based on serial clinical observations.

Twenty-four boys in 21 families were studied. Three families each have two boys with the disease. All of the index patients are male subjects; all have a clinical form of X-linked progressive muscular dystrophy which is thought to be typical of this disease. This appears to be a homogeneous group of patients; all with the same disease.

Although the families represent a wide spectrum of socioeconomic and educational status, most appeared to be in the lower middle class, with high school education the rule among the parents. These findings and our observations suggested that communication skills among these parents are well enough developed to insure reasonable understanding.

73

## Methods

The survey was conducted primarily by a professional medical social worker who was aided by a physician. Although some of the interviews were completed in the clinic at the time of a visit, the majority were accomplished in the patients' homes. All basic points were covered in each interview but the conversation was generally informal. Both parents were invited to participate. Questions relative to the economic status of the family, the level of self-care at which the patient functioned, and the ability of the patient to walk were followed by questions about the genetics of the disease. Information about the conception of children following the diagnosis of muscular dystrophy was requested, and the parents were asked what they knew about the possibility of similarly affected children resulting from subsequent pregnancies. Knowledge of the possible presence of the carrier state in sisters and whether brothers could be carriers of the disease were explored. All questions were asked in several ways to determine, if possible, the exact state of knowledge. The source of information was requested, when known. Finally, the family was asked for knowledge of the prognosis; specifically how long they expected the boy to live. Attitudes of the parents regarding the need for school and for special vocational efforts were reviewed.

Throughout the interview, information was provided where it was found lacking if the interviewer felt that the mother or father seemed receptive to learning more about the disease. Frequently, this information was confirmed and supplemented by the physician.

## Results

Table 1 shows that six children were conceived after the diagnosis was made in the index patient. All were born into separate families. The three boys have muscular dystrophy.

Table 1.—Initiation of Completed Pregnancies Related to Parents' Knowledge of Diagnosis

| Time of Conception | Sex of Siblings | | |
|---|---|---|---|
| | Boys | Girls | Total |
| Before diagnosis known | 27 | 21 | 48 |
| After diagnosis known | 3 | 3 | 6 |
| | | | 54 |

Table 2.—Parents' Genetic Knowledge Related to Source of Patient's Diagnosis

| Source of Diagnosis | Genetic Knowledge | | | |
|---|---|---|---|---|
| | Accurate | Inac-curate | None | Total |
| Author's clinic | 3 | 1 | 3 | 7 |
| Private doctor | 3 | 4 | ... | 7 |
| Other clinics | 2 | 4 | ... | 6 |
| Health department | 1 | ... | ... | 1 |
| Total | 9 | 9 | 3 | 21 |

Table 3.—Parent's Knowledge of Prognosis and Source of Information *

| | Complete | Incomplete |
|---|---|---|
| Author's clinic | 2 | 3 |
| Other medical facilities | 9 | 2 |
| Reading | 4 | ... |
| Friends and relatives | 1 | 1 |
| Own experience | 2 | 5 |

* Several families received information from multiple sources.

Whether the girls are carriers is not presently known. In four families, the index patient is the only child. It could not be determined why only six completed pregnancies were initiated after the diagnosis was made. In all cases, several years had elapsed after diagnosis, but fear of the disease per se was *stated* to be the cause in only two families. Illness, physical disability, death, divorce, and financial worries were all listed by one or more families, but no consistent pattern of reasoning was determined.

All of the families state that they plan no additional children, and nine parental pairs stated a present fear of additional children with the disease. The discrepancies between past performance, past attitudes, and present attitude are unexplained but suggest that accurate data regarding conception or its prevention are not easy to obtain. In only one family could a bias against artificial birth control be detected.

Table 2 illustrates the level of genetic information detected in the 21 families regarding the probability of the disease appearing in a subsequent sibling. The knowledge was designated inaccurate if part of the requested information was incorrect or absent. In only nine of the 21 families could accurate information and understanding be ascertained. In the remainder the information was either inaccurate, incomplete, or absent. Particularly, information about the possible carrier state was frequently inaccurate.

Table 2 also indicates the source of the diagnosis for the 21 families compared with the genetic information which accompanied that diagnosis. How often this important information was not provided is emphasized.

Table 3 summarizes the parents' knowledge of the patient's prognosis correlated with the source of that information. Several families indicated multiple sources of information. Only 14 of the families had been told by the physician that this disease would shorten the patient's life. In one case, it was alleged that the life span would not be shortened. Table 3 illustrates the fact that the knowledge related to prognosis is frequently inadequate.

Only eight families seemed to appreciate a need for an educational program modified to meet the intellectual, physical, and emotional needs of the child. Fifteen families agreed that some vocational planning was indicated, but in no case had appropriate, imaginative planning been initiated.

### Comment

The data indicate that in this study population, information concerning the genetics and prognosis of progressive muscular dystrophy has not been fully and systematically shared with the patients' families. It is possible that in at least three cases, the implementation of the *then* available information could have prevented the birth of three boys with this disease. It is evident that there is poor understanding among these families in regard to the carrier state, that the true prognosis for these patients is not always clear to the families, and that realistic efforts at education and vocational training are seldom appreciated and implemented.

The reasons for failure are many. At least one possibility is the lack of clear responsibility among the several members of the clinic team. No clear responsibility for assuring complete understanding had been assigned to any member of the staff. It seems reasonable to assign this responsibility jointly to the social worker and to a physician on the clinic staff, preferably the clinic director. The social worker is trained to be very instrumental in detecting a lack of knowledge, as well as providing the physician supplementary information regarding the patient's feelings, the parents' attitudes, and their receptiveness to additional information. The social worker could, following the physician's explanation of the facts of the disease to the parents, logically supplement this information from time to time and could, on repeated visits, question the parents to be sure that accurate knowledge is established. The social worker and physician could help implement whatever action the parents might wish to take regarding contraception or identification of carriers. The same principles may be applicable in clinics dealing with any diseases having well established inheritance patterns.

Thus, the social worker acts as an extension of the physician, detecting needs, suggesting solutions, and providing the impetus for the physician to efficiently intervene, amplify, and explain under optimum circumstances. At a time when the development of nurse practitioners and other similar aides seems to be a reasonable way to extend the influence of the physician and thus mitigate the critical shortage of physicians, the same principle could be applied in a similar fashion by these new health workers.

In brief, the medical center clinic should serve as a model for the delivery of health care. We have demonstrated significant failure in one area and suspect that it may be common. We have also proposed at least one solution which can be implemented today. The general use of these principles in congenital cardiac clinics, neurology clinics, and many other similar activities, as teaching models, could have significant impact on the effectiveness of health care.

This investigation was supported in part by a grant from Muscular Dystrophy Associations of America, Inc.

## References

1. Tips RL, Lynch HT: Genetic counselling in a team setting. *Birth Defects* 4: 110-113, 1968.

2. Neser WB, Sudderth GB: Genetics and casework. *Social Casework* 46:22-25, 1965.

3. Schild S: The challenging opportunity for social workers in genetics. *Social Work* 11:22-29, 1966.

4. Cohen HJ, Molnar GE, Taft LT: The genetic relationship of progressive muscular dystrophy (Duchenne type) and mental retardation. *Develop Med Child Neurol* 10:754-765, 1968.

# FAMILY COUNSELING

EVA KRMPOTIC, M.D., CHARLES FIELDS, M.D.,
AND KATARINA SZEGO, M.T.

In Parts II and III of this series,[1,2] we discussed the syndromes caused by chromosome abnormalities. The present paper deals with counseling, the procedure in which the physician explains to the affected person or family the existing genetic abnormality, the prognosis for the patient and his family, and the probability of recurrence in future offspring. Counseling is an integral part of cytogenetics and, aside from the diagnosis, should be the major concern of the physician.

Three categories of families seek family counseling: 1) those who had an abnormal child and want to know the chances of recurrence; 2) those with repeated abortions, stillbirths, or infertility — in the last case the individual himself will usually seek counseling; 3) those families who for different reasons have misgivings about the possibility of abnormality in an offspring (e.g., advanced age of the mother, rubella infection, etc.).

The management of all congenital or chronic diseases involves counseling by the physician. He has to inform the patient about the nature of his illness and its prognosis, and instruct him on how to cope with his affliction, what foods or environmental hazards to avoid, etc.

Counseling in cytogenetics differs from this in four aspects:

1) In most cases of cytogenetic abnormalities, the syndrome includes congenital malformation, mental retardation or psychologic deviations, and the management of these problems requires special attention.

2) In some cases the disease is familial: the abnormal chromosome is transmitted from the parents to the offspring. Since the clinical signs are, as a rule, the same as in the non-familial type of the disease and since only chromosome studies can establish the difference, a cytogenetic diagnosis should be obtained in every case.

3) Cytogenetic disorders affect not only the patient but his whole family and future generations; thus, not only the patient and his close relatives but also the whole family has to be informed and assisted in understanding the genetic problems involved.

77

4)  Cytogenetic counseling should not include advice on how to handle the situation (i.e., whether to have or not to have children). The counselor should, however, make sure that the problems are correctly understood, so that the members of the family will be equipped to make a sensible decision.

The conditions related to cytogenetic disorders have been recognized only during the last decade. Medical cytogenetics is a fairly new discipline. Counseling, therefore, should be undertaken only by physicians who thoroughly understand the entire scope of the genetic disorder involved and are able to provide proper guidelines for the decisions of the family. The counselor should also be aware of the psychological effect of his disclosures and use great tact in his dealings with the family concerned.

The above four points, referred to as being specific to cytogenetic counseling, should be considered by the physician before he communicates with the patient or his family.

Ideally, genetic counseling should be done by the physician who re-ferred the patient to the cytogenetics laboratory. He is the physician whom the patient consulted; in most cases he will know the specific situation of the patient and his family, and should be in the best position to evaluate the psychological impact of the genetic facts to be disclosed. However, since the chromosomal syndromes have been relatively recently recognized, many physicians, though proficient in their own specialties, will not possess up-to-date information in the growing field of medical genetics, and especially in cytogenetics. If the referring physician does not feel competent in this field, he should ask the cytogeneticist to render the counseling service. In the latter case, the cytogeneticist should be a physician familiar with all aspects of cytogenetic disease.

With the improvement of laboratory techniques it has become possible to diagnose chromosome abnormalities during early pregnancy. Thus, genetic counseling in a broader sense can serve as a preventive measure that can help reduce the frequency of congenital malformations and mental retardation in newborns.

It is the purpose of this article to familiarize physicians with the problems involved in family counseling. We will list the most frequent causes of cytogenetic abnormalities, discuss the nature of the problems, outline the probability of recurrence and describe the criteria established for cytogenetically high risk pregnancies. We will also discuss briefly the technical aspects of counseling and give examples of possible misin-terpretation.

Syndromes caused by abnormal chromosomes are divided into those produced by autosomal and those produced by sex chromosome abnormalities. Since different counseling is needed for the two categories, each will be discussed separately.

## AUTOSOMAL CHROMOSOME ABNORMALITIES

The cytogenetic diagnosis and the main signs of these syndromes have been outlined in Part II of this series.[1]

### DOWN'S SYNDROME (ALSO CALLED MONGOLISM).

Although the extra No. 21 chromosome is the cause of the disease in all cases, the three cytogenetic variations of the disease, regular trisomy, translocation trisomy, and mosaic trisomy, must be considered in genetic counseling.

Regular trisomy 21 is caused during cell division by nondisjunction of chromosomes during meiosis or of chromatids during mitosis.

If nondisjunction of the No. 21 chromosomes occurs during meiosis, two abnormal gametes will result: one containing 24 chromosomes with two No. 21 chromosomes, the other containing 22 chromosomes without a No. 21 chromosome. The gamete with 22 chromosomes is, as a rule, not viable. When the gamete containing the 24 chromosomes is united with a normal germ cell containing 23 chromosomes, the resulting zygote will have a regular trisomy 21 with 47 chromosomes. The offspring will have 47 chromosomes in all cells and will show the clinical signs of Down's syndrome.

Regular trisomy 21 can be produced also after fertilization in a normal zygote by nondisjunction of the No. 21 chromosomes during the first cleavage. The cell containing 45 chromosomes (monosomy 21) will usually not be viable. The cell with 47 chromosomes will divide further and all cells will contain 47 chromosomes.

The incidence of regular trisomy 21 and of all other chromosome abnormalities in which the cause of the disease is nondisjunction of an autosome is directly proportional to the age of the mother and increases significantly in mothers past 35 years of age.

Penrose and Smith[3] studied the maternal age distribution in Down's syndrome in 11 different countries and found a mean maternal age of 34.4 years. Paternal age does not seem to play a role. This is probably due to the fact that at the time of fertilization the age of the female germ cell is practically identical with the age of the mother, whereas the paternal germ cell is only a few weeks or months old.

In the United States alone about 7000 babies with Down's syndrome are born yearly. The frequency is 1 in 600-700 live births. Eighty percent of all cases are born to mothers older than 35.[2] One in 1000-2000 babies born to mothers between 19-29 years of age have Down's syndrome. The incidence doubles in the age group from 29-34, and becomes fivefold in the next five-year age group. In the maternal age group of 39-44, one out of 100-200 live births is affected; and in ages over 44 one out of 30-50.[4]

In translocation trisomy 21, the second cytogenetic type of Down's syndrome, the maternal age is of no significance. The translocation chromosome can be transmitted from generation to generation. If it becomes the cause of translocation trisomy 21, the disease is called familial Down's syndrome. Translocation trisomy 21 can arise also de novo and be present in the mongoloid offspring without carrier parents.

The most frequent chromosomes involved in translocation of the extra No. 21 chromosome are those of groups D13-15 and G21-22. In these cases the translocation chromosome is the result of the centric fusion of the long arms of a D13-15 or a G21-22 group chromosome and of the extra No. 21 chromosome.

Although the translocation chromosome represents a structural chromosome abnormality, the carrier of such a chromosome will be phenotypically normal if his or her chromosome complement contains no extra chromosome material. This type of translocation is called a balanced translocation in contrast to unbalanced translocation in which extra chromosome material is present, and the affected individual will have a translocation trisomy. Unfortunately, the detection of a carrier parent is preceded in most cases by the birth of an affected child to a member of the family. If one of the parents is a carrier, the risk of mongolism is 1 in 4 pregnancies. If one of the parents is a carrier of a D/21 translocation chromosome the following four possibilities should be considered: the haploid germ cells may contain 1) normal D13-15 and G21-22 chromosomes; 2) the D/21 translocation chromosome but no normal No. 21 chromosome; 3) the D/21 translocation chromosome and the normal No. 21 chromosome; 4) the normal D13-15 chromosomes but no No. 21 chromosome. After fertilization by a normal spermatozoon in a case where the mother is the carrier, or after fertilization of a normal egg, in a case where the father is the carrier, the resulting zygote may have the following: 1) a normal chromosome complement of 46 chromosomes resulting in a normal child; 2) a chromosome complement of 45 chromosomes resulting in a translocation carrier like the carrier parent; 3) a translocation trisomy 21 with 46 chromosomes resulting in a mongoloid child; 4) a monosomy 21 with 45 chromosomes, resulting, as a rule, in abortion.

There is some evidence that the D chromosomes involved in translocations may be nonrandomly selected. Thirty-four out of 39 cases studied by autoradiographic techniques were 14/21 translocations, while 5 were 15/21 translocations. No 13/21 translocations were found.[5]

In cases of 21/21 translocation the genetic prognosis is different. Since in this translocation the homologous No. 21 chromosomes are involved, one germ cell will, after meiosis, contain the translocation chromosome, and the other will lack the No. 21 chromosome.

If the germ cell containing the translocation chromosome is united with a normal germ cell, the offspring will have a translocation trisomy 21/21 and the clinical signs of Down's syndrome. If the germ cell without a No. 21 chromosome is involved in fertilization, the offspring will have monosomy 21 which, as a rule, will result in miscarriage. Families where one of the parents is a carrier of a 21/21 translocation thus cannot have normal children. Although the 21/21 translocation is the most serious type of translocation as far as future children are concerned, it is not a problem of the whole family because these translocations occur de novo in the parents and there is no further familial transmission of the translocation chromosome. Unfortunately, when a G/21 translocation is detected either in a carrier or the patient, the possibility of determining whether the translocation chromosome is a 21/21 or 21/22 translocation is limited with the present techniques. Autoradiography used for identification of the abnormal sex chromosomes or D group chromosomes proved to be useless in the identification of G group chromosomes. Only the pedigree of the family can provide the information needed to identify the chromosomes involved; if a couple had a normal child and one of the parents is a carrier of a G/21 translocation chromosome, the other G chromosome must be a No. 22. The probabilities of having a normal child, or a translocation carrier, or a translocation trisomy, or a monosomy 21 (as a rule not viable) are the same in a 21/22 translocation carrier as they are in a parent with D/21 translocation, namely 1:1:1:1.

The 21/21 translocation chromosome causes the same clinical syndrome as a No. 21 isochromosome. In both cases the chance for an affected child is 100% if either of the parents is a carrier. Recently, Hecht et al.[6] suggested that the pairing relationships of chromosomes during first meiosis are different in 21/22 and 21/21 translocations. Meiotic studies, however, have their limitations because of the usually poor quality of the meiotic chromosome preparation and the small number of cells in meiosis present in testicular and especially in ovarian biopsies. In addition, such a study in males is feasible only in sexually mature individuals in whom germ cell production is active. With improvement of techniques, meiotic studies should become valuable tools in family counseling.

Although the cause of translocation is unknown, it is reasonable to assume that this structural chromosome abnormality is the result of chromosome breaks and subsequent centric fusion of the involved chromosomes. Double chromosome abnormalities (Fig. 1) present in a single person suggest that the same environmental factor may cause either structural or numerical chromosome abnormalities or both. The phenomenon of structural and numerical abnormalities within a single cell population may indicate also that structural abnormality in a cell favors subsequent nondisjunction.

About 60% of all cases of maternal-age-related Down's syndrome are estimated to be caused by nondisjunction of the No. 21 chromosome.

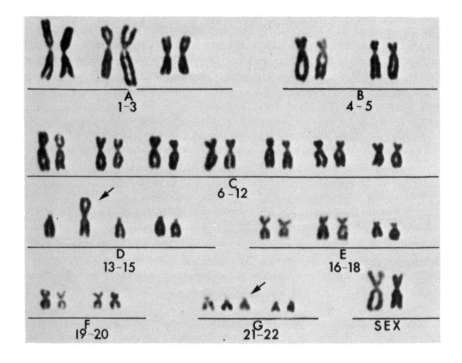

**FIGURE 1**

Double chromosome abnormality in a girl: 46, XX, 2D-, t(13q14q)+, 21+. Arrows point to the abnormal chromosomes.

Of the remaining 40%, 5-10% are due to translocation trisomy 21 and less than half of those are caused by familial translocation.

Nondisjunction during the first cleavage has been discussed under regular trisomy 21. If nondisjunction of the No. 21 chromosomes occurs during the second cleavage in one of the two cells, three cell types will result: the normal cell will have daughter cells with a normal chromosome complement of 46; one of the daughter cells of the cell with nondisjunction will have 47 chromosomes with trisomy 21; the other will have 45 chromosomes with monosomy 21 (cells, as a rule, not viable). Accordingly, the cells of the developing embryo will show two chromosome patterns: some cells will have 46 chromosomes, the others will have 47 chromosomes. The cytogenetic diagnosis for this condition is mosaic trisomy 21.

Mosaic trisomy 21 originates always in the offspring. The patients show usually the same clinical signs as in regular trisomy 21, although they may appear in milder form. The number of cells with trisomy 21 may be low in some cases, and this may make the diagnosis difficult. The offspring of a person with mosaic trisomy 21 will have either regular trisomy 21 because of secondary nondisjunction during gametogenesis if the fertilized germ cell contains the trisomy, or will be normal. On the basis of dermatoglyphic deviations, Penrose[7] estimated that 11% of all cases of trisomy 21 were caused by secondary nondisjunction, 10% occurring in the ova and 1% in the spermatozoa. Maternal age does not play a role in the etiology of these chromosome abnormalities.

Environmental factors such as X-ray radiation, virus infections, exposure to ultraviolet light, chemical poisons, fluoride content of the water, air pollution and even emotional stress in the mother were incriminated in the pathogenesis of nondisjunction or structural chromosome abnormalities (reciprocal translocation, centric fusion, isochromosome formation). Actually, we do not know yet what causes these chromosome abnormalities. The most recent hypothesis on the etiology of nondisjunction has been proffered by LeJeune. According to his theory premature rupture of the graafian follicle and subsequent fertilization of the immature oocyte causes trisomy 21 in the offspring, and may be the result of hormonal changes in advanced age of the mother. This theory, as all the others, has not been proven.

Whereas Down's syndrome has been known as a definite clinical entity long before trisomy 21, its cytogenetic cause, was discovered, most of the other congenital abnormalities were not recognized as distinct disease entities until their connection with certain chromosome aberrations had been established. Among them, trisomy 18 and trisomy 13 are the most important autosomal chromosome abnormalities.

In 1960, Edwards and his co-workers[8] described a patient with multiple congenital defects and trisomy of a group E16-18 chromosome. Autoradiographic studies identified the chromosome as a No. 18 chromosome.

An incidence of about 1 in 3000-5000 live births was established for this syndrome. The life expectancy for most of these patients is only a few months, although a small number have survived for more than two years. There are three times more females born with this chromosomal defect than males, possibly because the two similar sex chromosomes in the female (XX) provide a better balance for the extra chromosome. In Edwards' syndrome as in Down's syndrome, the three cytogenetic variations (regular, translocation, and mosaic trisomy) should be considered in family counseling. Advanced maternal age is again the most common known factor involved in the pathogenesis of the disease. In a small percentage of cases reciprocal translocation in a carrier parent or secondary nondisjunction could be demonstrated.

## TRISOMY 13

Trisomy of the No. 13 chromosome is the cause of this disease, also called Patau's syndrome after Patau who established its cytogenetic nature.[9] The incidence is about 1 in 5000-10,000 live births; as trisomy 18, it occurs more frequently in females than in males. The rarity of this syndrome in the newborn population is probably due to early intrauterine death, in many cases so early that the miscarriage is not recognized as such.

The three different cytogenetic prototypes (regular, translocation, and mosaic trisomy 13) have been described. The most common balanced structural chromosome abnormality is believed to be the centric fusion translocation involving two D group chromosomes (1 in 1000). Non-random selection of the D group chromosomes has been suggested in these cases. Of 34 cases gathered by Rowley and Pergament,[5] 26 were 13/14, four 13/15, three 13/13 and only one was a 14/15 translocation. If the translocation carrier has a nonhomologous translocation of the No. 13 chromosome, the chances for an affected offspring are one in four. The actual number, however, is much smaller because of the previously mentioned nonviability of the conceptus. This hypothesis is supported by the report of Mary Lucas[10] in which a phenotypically normal woman with a D/D translocation (apparently 15/15) was described who had at least 13 unsuccessful pregnancies, all terminating in early miscarriages. She had no live-born children. It should be kept in mind that in cases of repeated abortions, balanced structural abnormality in one of the parents might be the causative factor.

The syndromes described thus far are caused by a supernumerary chromosome. In contrast, the cause of malformations in the Cat Cry syndrome is the deletion of chromosome material, specifically the loss of the short arm of a group B4-5 chromosome.

Other "deletion syndromes," such as deletion of the short or long arm of a No. 18 chromosome, or deletion of a No. 21 chromosome, and others have been described. The clinical signs in these syndromes are not constant. Most probably, the size of the deleted portion of the chromosome is responsible for the variations, although the individual genetic background may also play an important role in the phenotypic expression of the disease. Maternal age does not seem to be involved as an etiologic factor. If there is no familial transmission of a structurally abnormal chromosome, the chances for recurrence are relatively small.

Many other autosomal chromosome abnormalities may result in mental retardation or congenital malformations. A "funny-looking" face and two or more congenital malformations with a concurrent "slow" mental development could be indicators of a chormosomal basis of the abnormality. The cause may be a balanced translocation in one of the parents. In repeated abortions, an unbalanced translocation in the offspring should be considered among the possible causes.

In all these cases as in any other genetic disorder, a physical examination, laboratory studies, and a carefully-taken and well-evaluated family history should precede the genetic counseling.

The risk of recurrence of autosomal chromosome abnormalities in future offspring depends on the cytogenetic variation of the disease. If the abnormality is related to the age of the mother, the risk of recurrence is increased in any subsequent pregnancy. If the abnormality is of the familial type, the danger of recurrence has to be seriously considered, and every pregnancy in such a family should be regarded as genetically high risk. In sporadic cases in which neither the maternal age nor inheritance can be incriminated in the etiology of the disease, the risk of having another affected child is not greater, or not significantly greater, than in the general population.

## SEX CHROMOSOME ABNORMALITIES

So far, we have described the counseling aspects of genetic diseases caused by autosomal chromosome abnormalities.

The following syndromes are based on sex chromosome abnormalities, and the patients are seeking family counseling not only because of congenital malformations but even more often because of infertility, repeated abortions or stillbirths.

The diagnostic cytogenetic aspects of the prototypes of these diseases in females and males (Turner's and Klinefelter's syndromes, respectively) have been discussed in Part III of this series.

## TURNER'S SYNDROME

It is estimated that a sex chromosome abnormality is present in about one in 3000 female newborns. This is, however, only a small fraction of the real number of such abnormalities since spontaneous abortions are not taken into consideration. Data from abortus studies suggest that 95% of female embryos or fetuses with defective sex chromosomes will result in miscarriage.[11] Systematic chromosome studies should be made a part of the pathologic examination of specimens from spontaneous abortions.

Usually, sex chromosome abnormalities are not detected at birth, unless the signs (webbed neck, low hair line, low birth weight, or marked edema of hands and feet) suggest such an anomaly to a well-informed physician. Failure of normal development or abnormally low stature of the child may later arouse this suspicion. In late puberty, continuing juvenile appearance of the genitalia and absence of menstruation will finally bring the patient to the office of a physician. Personality changes, erroneously described by some authors as mental retardation, may often be present at that time. In most cases, psychological and psycho-social problems due to the apparent sexual immaturity are the basis for the strange and childish behavior.

Maternal age is not an important factor in the causation of the disease. In addition to nondisjunction in the ovum or nondisjunction during cleavages, nondisjunction during spermatogenesis and anaphase lag during oogenesis were incriminated in the pathogenesis. The chromosomal basis of the disease is one abnormal X chromosome; therefore, not only the complete lack of one X chromosome, but also the deletion of the short or long arm,[12] ring chromosome formation or an iso-X-chromosome will cause the clinical syndrome. Mosaicism with one clone having the numerical or structural abnormality described above will result in the same syndrome although in a milder form. The syndrome can be diagnosed easily and quickly in the laboratory.

Chromosome studies are becoming increasingly common tests in a well equipped clinical laboratory and can be requested from any cytogenetics laboratory situated close enough so a mailed blood specimen can be received within 48 hours. Even when a cytogenetics laboratory cannot be reached, examination of a buccal smear for the presence of Barr bodies or of a vaginal smear for the demonstration of estrogen deficiency will give an important insight into the nature of the disease; an elevated level of pituitary gonadotropins (FSH) will further strengthen the suspicion. In all those cases in which clinical and laboratory examinations point to a possible diagnosis of

Turner's syndrome, one should not hesitate to obtain confirmation of the diagnosis from a cytogenetics laboratory. Medical management with hormonal replacement therapy will induce the development of secondary sex characteristics and anovulatory menstrual bleeding, and will help to restore the psychological integrity of the patient. Naturally, such a patient will remain sterile because the gonadal dysgenesis is not influenced by the therapy, and the height of the patient will not increase either. Otherwise, with medical help and proper counseling, such a patient could lead a comparatively normal life and even a marriage is not impossible. It is important that the genetic counselor explain to the patient the facts about her sterility, so she does not expect to be able to bear children. If the counseling is premarital, the future husband should also be informed, since sterility is a legal ground for divorce in most of the states.

## KLINEFELTER'S SYNDROME

This is the prototype of the male sex chromosome abnormality XXY. The frequency is about 1 in 400 live male births. It is possibly the most frequent sex chromosome anomaly. It has been seldom found in chromosome studies on aborted material indicating that an XXY sex chromosome complement is far less deleterious to the embryo than an XO sex chromosome anomaly. It also explains the fact that about eight times as many male as female newborns with a sex chromosome abnormality survive.

The counseling problems in Klinefelter's syndrome deserve special attention. Most often these patients or their families seek medical advice in late puberty. The physical appearance, especially the large breasts and sparse pubic hair with a female distribution, and almost no facial hair will arouse the suspicion of some existing irregularity. In other cases, the attention of the family is concentrated on the "strange behavior" of the affected member. Mental deficiency, homosexuality, psychopathic behavior may be also "diagnosed." It is generally believed, however, that mental retardation is not a characteristic sign of the disease but is the effect of psychologic difficulties in adaptation. With adequate medical management (hormonal therapy and psychotherapy, if needed) very few, if any, of these patients would have to be in mental institutions. They could live a normal life, fulfilling their social and economic role in the community of men. Although, as a rule, they cannot have children, their sexual life can be satisfactory and a normal marital life can be expected.

The success of medical management depends, however, on early prepubertal diagnosis of the disease. If instituted at the time of early puberty, the substitutional hormone therapy will induce development of the secondary sex characteristics, and reduce the frustrations of a sexually underdeveloped individual, thus avoiding or at least alleviating psychological disturbances caused by these deficiencies.

This ultimate aim of a well programmed medical management cannot be reached if the diagnosis of a sex chromosome abnormality is made too late because no clinical signs have aroused suspicion of the disease prior to puberty. Sex chromatin surveys of all newborns or pre-school children is, therefore, the essential prerequisite of a successful medical management of patients with sex chromosome abnormalities.

Another sex chromosome abnormality (XYY), the so called "double Y syndrome," should be mentioned because criminal behavior, subnormal intelligence and antisocial attitudes appear to have some connection. The majority of these patients are unusually tall. So far, a causal relationship has not been proven and more intensive screening of the normal population will be necessary to come to a final conclusion.

In the "intersex conditions", chromosome analysis will reveal the true nature of the disease, although chromosome abnormalities are not involved in its causation. True hermaphrodites have the gonads of both sexes, either separately or combined as ovotestes. Naturally, the gonads do not have a normal structure or function in either case, and these individuals are sterile. The apparent sex chromosome pattern is XX or XX/XY. Phenotypically, the patients may be either male or female and the external genitalia are ambiguous. Early cytogenetic diagnosis, followed by corrective surgery, hormonal treatment and, if needed, psychotherapy can alleviate the condition and assure a more or less normal social and economic adjustment for the patient. In pseudohermaphrodites the phenotypic sex is the opposite of the genetic sex. The cause of the abnormality is an abnormal gene and abnormal enzyme; hormone production interferes with the normal sexual development. Again clinical and laboratory studies carried out on time, and a proper medical management will greatly benefit the patient.

PREVENTIVE MEASURES

Family counseling is becoming more and more important in preventive medicine. The syndromes discussed are all hereditary disorders and, at present, successful treatment is not available for them. Only family counseling based on prenatal diagnosis and, in positive cases, therapeutic abortions may help to reduce the incidence of congenital malformations and mental retardation. Although the procedure for prenatal diagnosis seems complicated, it is a laboratory technique that can be mastered in any good cytogenetics laboratory. By making the cytogenetic diagnosis before birth the uncertainty in a genetically high risk pregnancy will be reduced to zero. Genetic counseling in a broader sense should, therefore, include as a preventive measure screening of all pregnancies for those that are genetically high risk. Recently, a prenatal Birth Defect Prevention Center has been established under the auspices of the National Foundation — March of Dimes at the Johns Hopkins Medical Institutions where families apprehensive of having defective children are counseled. If the results of clinical and cyto-genetic examinations clearly indicate the presence of a serious incurable disease, a choice of therapeutic abortion is offered to the parents.

At Mount Sinai Hospital Medical Center we have been conducting a screening program since 1969. Counseling consists of the following pro-cedures:

Expectant mothers (not later than in the fourth month of pregnancy) are interviewed and asked to complete, with the assistance of medical or paramedical personnel, the questionnaire shown in Fig. 2. The questionnaire was designed so that it can be filled out in two or three minutes, yet will provide enough information for separating genetically high risk pregnancies from those that are genetically low risk. If the pregnancy is considered genetically high risk, a second interview is arranged, and, if indicated, amniocentesis is recommended. If performed, specimens are submitted to the cytogenetics laboratory and studied for chromosome abnormalities; other laboratory investigations are done as needed. The cytogenetic diag-nosis is then sent to the referring physician.

In general, we consider four main categories as cytogenetically high risk pregnancies.

1.   Advanced maternal age. Maternal age is recognized as an im-portant factor in the etiology of Down's syndrome and other trisomy syn-dromes. The chromosome abnormalities in various syndromes have been described above and the estimated risk within certain age groups indicated. If the maternal age is over 37, we consider the pregnancy as genetically high risk and amniocentesis is recommended.

2.   Familial chromosome abnormalities. Structural chromosome ab-normalities such as reciprocal translocations, iso-chromosomes, and centric-fusion translocations can be transmitted from generation to generation. The recognition of the carrier status in the parents is of great importance because of the high probability of congenital malformations in the offspring. If either of the parents is a carrier, the pregnancy should be regarded as genetically high risk, regardless of the age of the mother. Numerical chromosome abnormalities in one of the parents (e.g. trisomy 21, partial trisomies) should be always regarded as high risk for the offspring because of the possibility of secondary nondisjunction.

3.   Genes favoring nondisjunction. Independently of maternal age and chromosome translocations, a specific abnormal gene in either gamete may disturb the process of cell division and produce several different chromo-some abnormalities in the same family. About 10% of all cases of Down's syndrome are believed to be caused by the action of such a gene. In families

Name of Referring Physician: _____
                    Address: _____
                Telephone No. _____

Name of Person Completing This Questionnaire: _____

Name of Patient: _____

   1) Age: _____       Gravida: _____       Para: _____

   2) Date of last menstruation: _____     E. D. C.: _____

   3) Age of father of offspring: _____

   4) Ages of living children: _____
      If not living, dates of birth and death, and cause of death: _____
      _____
      _____

   5) Number and dates of abortions or stillbirths and their causes:*
      _____
      _____

   6) Acute diseases during present pregnancy:** _____
      _____

   7) Chronic diseases:** _____
      _____

   8) Any mental retardation or congenital malformation in family of mother or
      father of the offspring for the last three generations:
      _____
      _____

   9) If answer to 8) is yes, describe the disease and give diagnosis, if known:
      _____
      _____

---

*To be answered by the physician, if possible.
*Additional information of possible significance by the physician will be appreciated
(especially drugs, x-ray exposure during and three months prior to pregnancy).


## FIGURE 2

Questionnaire for pregnant women.

90

where two or more members have chromosome abnormalities, any pregnancy should be regarded as genetically high risk, regardless of the age of the mother. Tracing the family history back through three generations is of utmost importance.

4.   Environmental factors. Acute viral diseases (such as rubella and cytomegalovirus infections) of the mother within the first trimester of pregnancy are known teratogenic factors. Examination of the amniotic fluid during such infections showed chromosomal breaks in more than 20% of the cells. Therefore, in addition to viral studies of the amniotic fluid, chromosome analysis is an important supplement to the laboratory diagnosis of such infections. Large doses of X-ray irradiations during early pregnancy also have been incriminated as an etiologic factor of congenital malformations; if 20% or more cells from the amniotic fluid cultures show chromosomal breaks, the accumulated data justify the classification of such pregnancies as genetically high risk.

The technique used for culturing cells from amniotic fluid was outlined by Jacobson et al. [13] The laboratory technique for prenatal detection of chromosome abnormalities is as follows:

A few cubic centimeters of amniotic fluid are obtained by suprapubic amniocentesis after the thirteenth or fourteenth week of pregnancy. It should be kept in mind that amniocentesis is a minor surgical intervention and should be carried out by an experienced physician. It is important that the specimen reaches the cytogenetics laboratory within 24 hours.

The desquamated fetal and amniotic cells are obtained from the fluid by centrifuging the specimen. The cells are placed in a tissue culture bottle (T-15 flask), covered with appropriate medium (medium 199 supplemented with 20% fetal bovine serum, 1% glutamine, 1% folic acid, and antibiotics), and incubated at 37°C. After the cells have grown to a full sheet, they are subcultured and after the subcultures have grown out to a full sheet, the procedure for obtaining metaphases from fibroblasts is applied. Cells with well distinguishable chromosome spreads are examined and photographed. Finally, the chromosomes are arranged into karyotypes for the cytogenetic diagnosis.

Before the final diagnosis is made, the cytogeneticist has to make sure that the fetal cells have not undergone transformation in tissue culture, and that the prepared karyotypes reflect the true chromosome complement of the fetal cells.

To illustrate the importance of these statements we will describe a family which was referred to us for family counseling. In this family, the father's brother had a child with Down's syndrome. The father also had

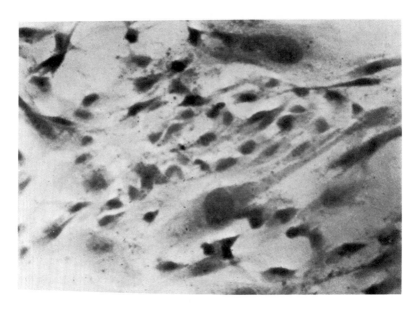

FIGURE 3

Cells from amniotic fluid grown in tissue culture.

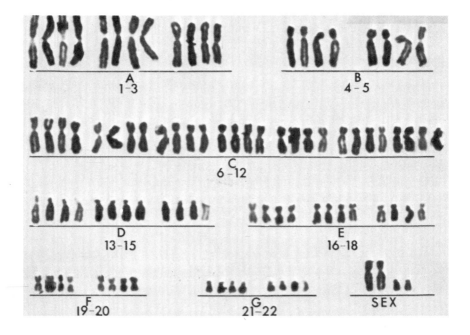

FIGURE 4

Karyotype of a tetraploid cell from tissue culture shown above.

such a child from his first marriage. Chromosome studies were done on the blood of the fathers and in both cases no abnormality was found. The affected child from the first marriage of the propositus' father died at an early age. The other affected child has been institutionalized and no chromosome study could be done. Since in both cases the mothers were less than 30 years old, advanced maternal age as predisposing factor to nondisjunction could be excluded. However, the present pregnancy was considered genetically high risk because of the possibility that "genes favoring nondisjunction" were present in this family, and amniocentesis was performed. A cytogenetic diagnosis could not be made from tissue culture cells from the first passage because of the relatively few metaphases present. For the following two to three weeks, very slow growth, if any, was observed in the tissue culture. Then, suddenly, the cells started to grow, doubling in less than 24 hours, so that subcultures had to be done practically every 48 hours (Fig. 3). Chromosome studies at that time showed tetraploidy or near tetraploidy of cells (from 38 metaphase spreads examined and photographed, not a single cell showed a normal chromosome complement) (Fig. 4). Because of the growth pattern, a transformation of the cells in tissue culture was suspected, excluding a conclusive diagnosis. A second amniocentesis was not feasible, since at that time the pregnancy was already advanced. On full term, a normal six-pound, ten-ounce, twenty-inch-long baby boy was born and the chromosome studies of the peripheral blood and skin cultures of the newborn revealed a normal male chromosome complement (Fig. 5).

Mycoplasma are fairly common contaminants in tissue culture and, although they will not interfere with the multiplication of cells for a few passages, they will cause chromosomal breaks. Since chromosomal breaks are important in counseling, it should be emphasized that the tissue cultures from cells obtained from the amniotic fluid should be handled under absolutely sterile conditions. When chromosomal breaks are studied, precautions against mycoplasma contamination should be sought in addition to precautions against bacterial and fungal contaminations, i.e. a mask should be worn during handling of the tissue culture.

Although chromosome studies from amniotic fluid do not present any difficulties to a good cytogenetics laboratory and diagnostic errors should not be encountered, these studies are time consuming, taking three to five weeks. The techniques are being further investigated to reduce the time needed for such a study and to make it ultimately possible to offer a diagnosis within 7 to 10 days.

The cytogenetic diagnosis is given by the cytogeneticist to the referring physician who will decide whether he or the cytogeneticist should assume the role of counselor. If the referring physician does the counseling, he should always remember that his function is only counseling and not

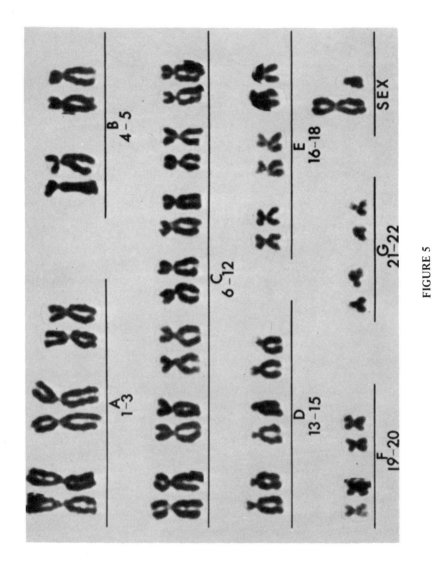

**FIGURE 5**

46, XY. Normal male karyotype of a cell obtained from the skin culture of the newborn baby.

directing the decisions of the family involved. He should translate the cyto-genetic diagnosis into understandable information but the decision whether or not to take any therapeutic action should rest with the prospective parents.

## REFERENCES

1. Krmpotic, E., Uy, E., and Meeker, D.: Medical cytogenetics. Part II. Autosomal chromosome abnormalities. The Chicago Med. Sch. Quart. 27:98 (Winter), 1968
2. Krmpotic, E., Uy, E., and Szego, K.: Medical cytogenetics. Part III. Sex chromosome abnormalities and autoradiography of human chromosomes. The Chicago Med. Sch. Quart. 27:125 (Spring), 1968
3. Penrose, L.S. and Smith, G.F.: Down's Anomaly, Boston, Little, Brown and Company, 1966, p. 157
4. Reisman, L.E. and Matheny, A.P., Jr.: Counseling in Down's syndrome, In: Genetics and Counseling in Medical Practice, St. Louis, The C.V. Mosby Company, 1969, Chapter 6, pp. 66-69
5. Rowley, J.D. and Pergament, E.: Possible non-random selection of D group chromosomes involved in centric-fusion translocations. Ann. Genet. 12:177, 1969
6. Hecht, F., Delay, M., Seely, J.R., and Stoddard, G.R.: Meiotic evidence in Down's syndrome for 21/21 chromosome translocation or isochromosome. J. Pediat. 76:298, 1970
7. Penrose, L.S.: Dermatoglyphics in mosaic mongolism and allied conditions, In: Genetics Today, Vol. 3, Oxford, Pergamon Press, 1965, p. 973
8. Edwards, J.H., Harnden, D.G., Cameron, A.H., Crosse, V.N., and Wolff, O.H.A.: A new trisomic syndrome, Lancet 1:787, 1960
9. Patau, K., Smith, D.W., Therman, E., Inhorn, S.L., and Wagner, H.P.: Multiple congenital anomaly caused by an extra autosome. Lancet 1:790, 1960
10. Lucas, M.: Translocation between both members of chromosome pair number 15 causing recurrent abortions. Ann. Hum Genet. 32:347, 1969
11. Carr, D.H.: Chromosome studies in spontaneous abortions. Obstet. Gynec. 26:308, 1965
12. Hecht, F., Jones, D.L., Delay, M. and Klevit, H.: Xq – Turner's syndrome: Reconsideration of hypothesis that Xp – causes somatic features in Turner's syndrome. J. Med. Genet. 7:1 1970
13. Jacobson, C.B. and Barter, R.H.: Intrauterine diagnosis and management of genetic defects. Am. J. Obstet. Gynec. 99:796, 1967

# Genetic Counseling

# (A Scientific Exhibit)

HENRY T. LYNCH, M.D.

GABRIEL M. MULCAHY, M.D.

ANNE J. KRUSH, M.S.

## Introduction

THERE is a worldwide need for genetic counseling which should be an integral part of any medical approach when hereditary factors are either suspected or actually proven. In 1964, the World Health Organization Expert Committee on Human Genetics[1] recommended increased training of medical personnel in medical genetics, with particular emphasis on genetic counseling. Again in 1968[2] it was emphasized that "education of the general practitioner in medical genetics is most important. Teaching should be given at both the preclinical and clinical levels of medical education. It is equally important that medical genetics be dealt with in postgraduate education in refresher courses."

Genetic specialty clinics are not the answer. Specifically, there are too few of these clinics to meet the pressing demands for counseling. Furthermore, we firmly believe that the responsibility for genetic counseling can be best fulfilled by the family doctor; he is often the family's closest confidant and is usually the individual most familiar with the manifestations of a particular genetic disease in a particular family. Since our approach to genetic counseling entails diagnosis of the patient and of his relatives at genetic risk, therapy, and prognosis, the continuity of the overall plan will be best assured when the family doctor provides this important service.

The purpose of this exhibit is to present a variety of commonly seen genetic counseling problems, the handling and disposition of which should naturally fall within the responsibilities of the family physician.[3-13]

*Section 1: History*

Section 1 depicts the history of genetics, beginning in Biblical times and lists scientific contributions which help to form the basis of medical genetics and which have been applied in modern times to genetic counseling. We have not listed present workers in the fields (Figs. 1 and 2). We call particular attention to the citation of hemophilia in Figure 1. An early account of genetic counseling for this disease is found in the Babylonian Talmud, in the second century, in the writings of Rabbi Judah, when he stated, "If she circumcised her first child and he died (as a result of bleeding from the operation), and a second one also died (similarly), she must not circumcise her third child." Subsequent Rabbinic Responsa differed only in interpretation of the number of repetitive events, i.e., deaths following circumcision, which would confirm a pattern and thus remove the deaths from the realm of mere chance. A clinical example of counseling of a hemophilic family from our files will be presented below.

*Section 2: Mendelian Inheritance*

This section illustrates several examples of classical Mendelian inheritance with genetic counseling implications. These include mandibulofacial dysostosis (inherited as an autosomal dominant), xeroderma pigmentosum (inherited as an autosomal recessive), hemophilia (inherited as a sex-linked recessive, to be discussed below), and vitamin D-resistant rickets (inherited as a sex-linked dominant).

## Hemophilia
### (Sex-Linked Recessive)

Severe guilt in this family was linked to overprotectiveness by mothers with hostility and rejection by some of the husbands who married into a hemophilia family. Affected children rebelled and "flirted" with danger to combat overprotective parents.

Misconceptions centered about "skipping generations" through unaffected but "carrier" females.

Genetic counseling permitted catharsis with surfacing of anxieties and subsequent alleviation of "blame" for this disease. The counselor fostered development of understanding of underlying rebelliousness of children and the need for normal childhood activities.

A detailed explanation was given of the significance of the carrier state in women with disclosure of risk of hemophilia to 50 percent of male progeny and of carrier state to 50 percent of female progeny of carrier mothers.

*Section 3: Cytogenetics*

This section includes illustrations of several cytogenetic anomalies including Down's

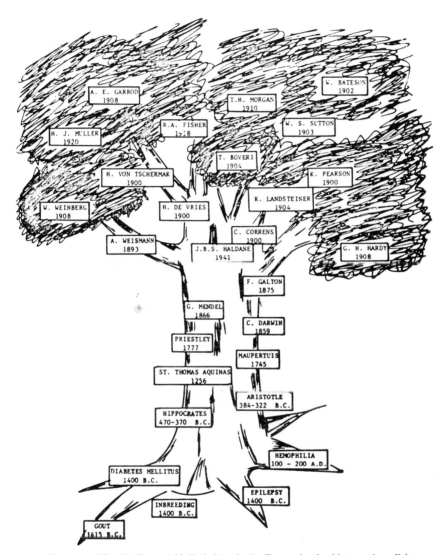

Figure 1. "Family Tree of Medical Genetics." Events in the history of medicine and genetics which have laid the groundwork for modern medical genetic counseling.

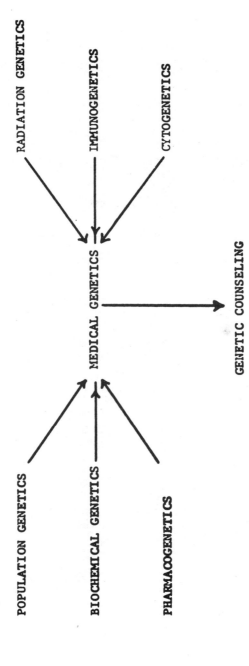

Figure 2. Interaction of specialty areas of medical genetics which collectively carry important implications for genetic counseling.

100

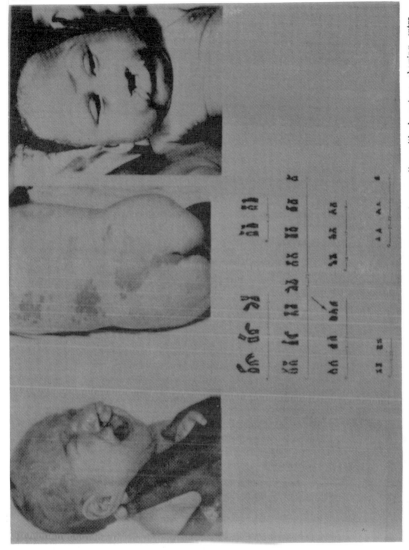

**Figure 3.** Baby with D-trisomy syndrome showing multiple congenital anomalies with karyotype showing extra chromosome in one of the members of the 13-15 groups.

101

syndrome, Cri-du-chat syndrome, Turner's syndrome, and D-trisomy (Fig. 3), to be discussed below.

### Clinical Indications for Chromosomal Analysis

1. Infants and children with mental retardation or congenital anomalies, consistent with altered chromosomal number, structure, or suspected chromosomal mosaicism.
2. Sterility and infertility problems.
3. Differential diagnosis of intersex.
4. Psychiatric symptoms with medicolegal implications in males (XYY).
5. Problems involving translocation chromosomes and familial occurrences of congenital abnormalities and/or mental retardation.
6. Repeated abortions.
7. Assessment of chromosomal damage due to virus, x-ray, or chemicals.
8. Hematology problems, as Philadelphia chromosome in chronic myelogenous leukemia.
9. Rare conditions such as Bloom's syndrome and Fanconi's anemia, in which chromosomal breakage may occur.

Cytogenetic studies are helpful when discernible chromosomal abnormalities of number or structure are present. In most genetic diseases, however, although mutations at the level of the gene no doubt occur, these are far too subtle for direct visual detection with current techniques of chromosomal analysis.

In genetic counseling we use karyotypes as an additional instructional tool for our patients so that they may better comprehend the biological significance of t h e chromosomal abnormalities. This o f t e n

102

Table 1

SOME DISORDERS OF ABNORMAL CHROMOSOMAL CONSTITUTION

| Condition | Significance to Individual | Significance to Family |
|---|---|---|
| Down's syndrome | Mental retardation. Associated congenital anomalies. High risk of leukemia. | 1. Sporadic, related to advanced maternal age.<br>2. Familial, some due to trans-location chromosome in cells of parent. |
| D trisomy | Death usually occurs in neo-natal period. | Generally sporadic. |
| E trisomy | Death in infancy is expected. | Generally sporadic. |
| Cri-du-chat syndrome (partial deletion of short arm of B group chromosome) | Mental retardation. Usually early death. | Generally sporadic. |
| Klinefelter's syndrome(XXY) | Alteration in habitus (eunuchoid-ism); mentality normal or sub-normal. Sterility. | Generally sporadic. |
| Turner's syndrome (XO) | Congenital abnormalities, infan-tile genitalia, short stature, sterility; favorable response to estrogen. | Generally sporadic. May be a familial auto-immune factor. |
| Triple X syndrome (XXX) | Mental retardation common. May have sterility problem. | Generally sporadic. |
| XYY syndrome | Possible relationship to aggres-sive criminal behavior. Full significance of karyotype un-certain. | Generally sporadic. |

minimizes attendant guilt feelings.

Table 1 lists some of the major disorders of abnormal chromosomal constitution, and gives a synopsis of their significance to both the affected individual and his family. The following discussion provides clinical details concerning one of these cytogenetic disorders, D-trisomy.

### D-Trisomy

In D-trisomy, a chromosome in the 13-15 group is triply rather than doubly represented, as a result of nondisjunction in parental gametogenesis. Manifestations of this syndrome include: microcephaly and defects of the skull, microphthalmia, low set or malformed ears, hemangiomas over the body, micrognathia, midline cleft of lip and palate, congenital cardiac and renal lesions, hypotonia, polydactyly, syndactyly, retroflexed thumbs, "rocker bottom" feet, abnormal dermatoglyphic patterns, severe mental retardation, and apneic seizures. Gross cerebral defects, particularly arhinencephalia, are present, perhaps accounting for this syndrome sometimes being confused with anencephaly (unassociated with a chromosomal defect). Infants do not usually survive beyond the first year of life.

*Section 4: Special Problems in Genetic Counseling*

Some of the problems posed by the presence of hereditary diseases within a kindred include:

1.  *Early hereditary death* as occurred in 3 siblings with cystinosis.

2.  *Empirical risk problems,* i.e., diseases with an increased incidence in families, but which do not follow simple Mendelian inheritance patterns. For instance, in breast

cancer the risk for women in the general population is approximately 5 percent. If a first degree relative has breast cancer, however, the risk is three-fold greater (approximately 17 percent).

3. *Scapegoating and community rejection* — often suffered by patients with grotesque phenotypes. Depicted is a family with myotonia dystrophica whose affected members were prejudged as being "stupid, sleepy, and disinterested" in social activities, when in fact the stigmata of this disease, ptosis, facial drooping, and profound muscle weakness, were responsible for conveying this impression.

4. *Medicolegal problems in teratology.* Congenital abnormalities discovered at birth cause anguish and may occasionally arouse hostility toward the physician, who may be accused of being "responsible" because of alleged neglect, sometimes leading to a malpractice suit. Studies must involve a careful survey for drugs, viruses, spirochetes, protozoa, anoxia, and other environmental teratogens during embryogenesis, as well as cytogenetic and genetic abnormalities.

5. *Adoption problems.* A married couple incapable of conception may wish to consider adoption. Studies have shown that adopted children usually adjust as well socially and emotionally as children born to natural parents. Collaboration of physician, social agency, and attorney is the preferred practice in adoptions.[14] Interests of the child are paramount. Therefore, the physician should discourage "b l a c k market" adoptions (an unauthorized agency selling the child to adopting parents) and independent placements ("gray market").

6. *Amniocentesis and prenatal diagnosis.*

a. *Rh incompatibility* — spectrophotometric measurements of pigment in amniotic fluid tend to indicate the status of the fetus.

b. *Sex determination* — Presence (female) or absence (male) of sex chromatin (Barr) bodies enables one to make a prediction of fetal sex.

c. *Cytogenetic abnormalities* — such as Down's syndrome, which is more likely to be diagnosed with advanced maternal age. Some have performed therapeutic abortions on the basis of chromosomal analysis of amniotic cells. This is highly controversial, of course, dependent as it is on the ethical and religious views of the individual concerned, and applicable statutes. Parents should be advised to consult the clergyman of their choice when faced with this type of decision.

d. *Biochemical studies* — Amniotic cells may be cultured in search of such aberrations as metachromasia which is associated with the mucopolysaccharidoses and cystic fibrosis; enzyme deficiencies, such as galactosemia, and homocystinuria; and cytoplasmic inclusions such as are found in Chediak-Higashi syndrome.

7. *Reassurance* is an exceedingly important phase of genetic counseling. It is essential to ascertain whether a particular disease is inherited or acquired. This problem may sometimes be resolved through careful ascertainment of family history since certain acquired diseases may mimic hereditary disorders (phenocopy). Occasionally the phenocopy may be more serious than the true hereditary form. An example is the Pelger-Huet anomaly, which is inherited as

an autosomal dominant and is characterized by faulty segmentation and condensation of granulocytic leukocytes. There is an acquired nongenetic phenocopy of this defect which occurs in such myelopathies as acute leukemia, chronic myelogenous leukemia, and myeloid metaplasia.

*Case History:* A physician underwent periodic screening physical and laboratory examinations offered to all physicians at annual medical meetings. His peripheral blood smears were "normal" until his most recent examination when a diagnosis of Pelger-Huet anomaly was made. Knowing only that the acquired form was associated with hematopoietic malignancies, he b e c a m e alarmed and sought the counsel of a hematologist colleague who informed him that there is a genetic form which is benign, and that this should be searched for to preclude the more ominous preleukemic state. The defect was subsequently identified in the proband's sibling and four of this sib's children, as well as in two of his own four children. Thus the patient was reassured that his was the benign or hereditary form of the Pelger-Huet anomaly (Fig. 4). (Acknowledgment is extended to Harry Hynes, M.D., and Michael Hogan, B.A., for providing the above history).

*Section 5: Preventive Medicine and Genetic Counseling*

1. *Xeroderma pigmentosum (xdp).* Since preventive measures for xdp involve avoidance of exposure to sun, genetic counseling must be concerned with the practical and psychological aspects of coping with this problem. Instilling a positive attitude toward self-care and self-protection is mandatory. Provision of protected areas for play and encouragement of participation in evening and indoor sports are also important.

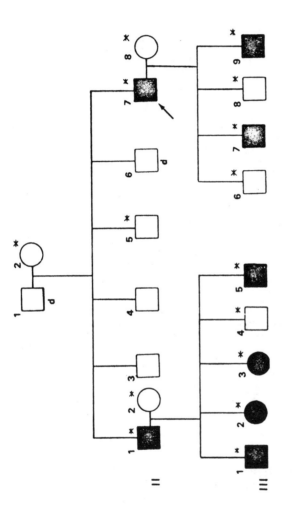

LEGEND

■ or ● MALE OR FEMALE c̄ PELGER-HUET ANOMALY

□ or ○ MALE OR FEMALE UNAFFECTED

↗ PROBAND

d DIED

* INDIVIDUAL EXAMINED

Figure 4. Pedigree of family with the hereditary form of the Pelger-Huet anomaly showing classical autosomal dominant inheritance.

2. *Familial polyposis coli* is inherited in an autosomal dominant manner. Forty percent of affected patients have cancer when the diagnosis is first made. Soberingly, virtually a 100 percent cure could be accomplished if colectomy were performed early in life prior to cancer transformation.

3. *Bronchogenic carcinoma.* There is an increased risk of this disease in cigarette smokers, but the risk becomes far greater in those individuals with a first degree relative who has a diagnosis of lung cancer. Their risk is 14-fold greater than for smokers in the general population.

4. *Diabetes mellitus.* This is a genetic disease, though the mode of inheritance is not clear. Genetic counseling is directed toward relatives at risk who are advised to control obesity, restrict saturated fats in their diet, and undergo periodic evaluation of blood sugar level.

5. *Rh factor and hemolytic disease of the newborn.* Control of hemolytic disease of the newborn due to an Rh problem can be achieved through administration of anti-Rho (Anti D) Immunoglobulin G (RhoGAM) to Rh negative mothers within 72 hours following each delivery of an Rh positive infant and each miscarriage. This will prevent the mother from forming Rh antibodies to those Rh positive rbc's t h a t might have crossed the placenta. Therefore, hemolytic disease of the newborn can be prevented in subsequent pregnancies. If the mother is already sensitized to the Rh factor, administration of anti-Rho is of no value and on that account, other measures, such as intrauterine transfusion and exchange transfusion, are indicated in treatment of the affected infant.

## Section 6: Summary

1. Approximately one third of all diseases have a genetic etiology.

2. Genetic counseling is an integral part of the total management of patients and their families with known or suspected genetic disease.

3. Not only because of an acute shortage of professional genetic counselors, but also because of his knowledge of the medical history of family complexes, the family physician must assume the responsibility for genetic counseling.

4. The person seeking advice should receive a clear estimate of the risk of hereditary transmission of the disease. If possible, the risk estimate should be given by the family physician who is in constant touch with the family and its problems; he can often give helpful guidance that takes into account many personal and social factors in addition to purely genetic considerations. He should be alert to the emotional problems that may be troubling his patients.

5. More counseling services should be established, especially in regions where infectious disease and nutritional disorders are being brought under control and understanding of the relative importance of hereditary disorders is increasing, and in areas where genetic disorders have always constituted a serious public health problem.

6. This exhibit focuses upon the medical milieu in which genetic counseling serves. Genetic counseling is based on relatively few genetic principles; it demands compassionate concern and an empathetic listening ear.

We express appreciation to Lillian Lockhart, M.D., and Charles C. Thomas, Publisher, for permission to use some of the illustrative material above, taken from the book, *Dynamic Genetic Counseling for Clinicians,* edited by Henry T. Lynch, M.D.

### References

1. Human Genetics and Public Health, Expert Committee on Human Genetics, No. 282, WHO Techn Rep Ser, 1964.

2. Genetic Counseling: Third Report of the WHO Expert Committee on Human Genetics, No. 416, WHO Techn Rep Ser, 1969.

3. Lynch, H. T.: Dynamic Genetic Counseling for Clinicians, New York, Charles C. Thomas, 1969, pp. 354.

4. Smith, G. S.; Lynch, H. T., and McNutt, C. W.: The "whole family" concept in clinical genetics. Amer J Dis Child 107:67-76, 1964.

5. Lynch, H. T.; Krush, T. P.; Krush, A. J., and Tips, R. L.: Psychodynamics of early hereditary deaths. Amer J Dis Child 108:605-610, 1964.

6. Lynch, H. T.; Krush, T. P.; Krush, A. J., and Tips, R. L.: Psychological variations in patients with gonadal dysgenesis (Turner's syndrome): report of two cases — role of the medical genetics counselor. J Lancet 86:340-344, 1966.

7. Lynch, H. T.; Tips, R. L., and Krush, A. J.: Psychodynamics in a chronic debilitating hereditary disease: myotonia dystrophica. Arch Gen Psychiat 14:153-157, 1966.

8. Lynch, H. T.; Tips, R. L.; Krush, A. J., and Magnuson, C. W.: Family centered genetic counseling and the medical genetics clinic. Nebraska Med J 50:155-159, 1965.

9. Lynch, H. T.; Anderson, D. E.; Krush, A. J., and Mukerjee, D.: Cancer, hereditary, and genetic counseling: xeroderma pigmentosum. Cancer 20:1796-1801 (October) 1967.

10. Lynch, H. T.: Practical aspects of the family history, genetics and genetic counseling: cancer. Nebraska Med J 53:6-11 (January) 1968.

11. Lynch, H. T., and Krush, A. J.: Heredity, emotions and cancer control. Postgrad Med 43:134-138 (February) 1968.

12. Lynch, H. T., and Krush, A. J.: Genetic counseling and cancer: implications for cancer control. Southern Med J 61:265-269 (March) 1968.

13. Krush, A. J.; Krush, T. P., and Lynch, H. T.: Psycho-social factors in a family with a disfiguring genetic fault Psychosomatics 6:391-396, 1965.

14. Adoption of Children, Committee on Adoption, American Academy of Pediatrics, Evanston, Illinois, 1967.

# Inheritance

WAYNE H. FINLEY
SARA C. FINLEY

Biochemical genetics, population genetics, cytogenetics, genetic counseling, and their relation to clinical medicine were the main topics on the program of the International Seminar on Medical Genetics held at the Medical Center, University of Alabama in Birmingham, 31 August to 3 September 1966. Participants came from the United States, Sweden, Poland, Italy, France, Great Britain, and Canada. J. F. Volker (vice president for Birmingham Affairs and director of the Medical Center of the University of Alabama in Birmingham) welcomed the guests. Alice Chenoweth (chief, Program Services Branch, Children's Bureau, Washington) expressed the hope that the rapid advances in biochemistry and cytogenetics would lead to knowledge of practical importance in solving heredity problems.

A. Motulsky (Seattle) opened the session on biochemical genetics. Using the abnormal hemoglobins as a model, he pointed out that details of the relation of molecular structure to pathologic function are better understood in the case of the hemoglobinopathies than in many other genetic diseases. In discussing advances in pharmacogenetics, Motulsky pointed out that drug reactions may serve as models for the interaction of genetically determined biochemical variability and exogenous agents. Neither the genetic abnormality nor the drug alone causes difficulty but the administration of the drug to the genetically susceptible individual results in disease. In relation to the feasibility of biochemical screening for the detection of heterozygotes, he emphasized that screening for X-linked diseases is practically more important in family counseling than screening for heterozygotes in autosomal disease.

The second day of the meeting was devoted to population genetics, and L. L. Cavalli-Sforza (Pavia), in discussing the structure of human populations, indicated that interest in the epidemiological aspects may help us to understand the heterogeneity of genetic traits. He discussed in particular some of his findings with the Pygmies. In comparing data on Western Pygmies, Negroes, and Eastern Pygmies, Cavalli-Sforza concludes that the Western Pygmies are nearer to the Negroes that surround them than to the Bushmen, while the Eastern Pygmies are nearer to the Bushmen than to the Negroes. The tentative conclusion is that it is possible and perhaps even likely that the Pygmies and Bushmen formed originally a single group. In response

112

to the question, "Can one consider these Pygmies as a proto-African population?" Cavalli-Sforza says the answer is probably yes.

C. J. Witkop (Minneapolis) presented his group's medical and dental findings in the Brandywine Isolate, an inbred population of mixed Caucasian, Negro, and Amerindian ancestry. Its population of today represents a breeding isolate in which most marriage partners are selected among persons having one of fifteen surnames. It appears that the Brandywine Isolate owes its peculiar gene distribution largely to the founder effect. The phenotypic frequencies for dentinogenesis imperfecta and tyrosinase-positive albinism were the highest reported for any population, and the gene frequency for sickle-cell hemoglobin was the highest reported in a United States population. J. A. Böök (Uppsala) indicated that the genetical determinants in mental retardation are mostly specific major gene mutations or chromosome mutations. He also discussed the polygenic component of the variance in intelligence.

V. A. McKusick (Baltimore) discussed the ethnicity of disease in the United States, and pointed out that such studies are useful in diagnosis and management as well as for the design of screening programs. Diseases with relatively high frequency in four Amish groups that appear to represent separate demes include the Ellis-van-Creveld syndrome, hemolytic anemia associated with pyruvate kinase deficiency, hemophilia B, and autosomal recessive limb girdle muscular dystrophy. Familial dysautonomia is also being studied on a total ascertainment basis.

The third day was devoted to papers and discussion in cytogenetics and genetic counseling. J. Lejeune (Paris) discussed "Gene Dosage Effects." Excess or missing chromosomal material which is associated with abnormal clinical findings was the basis for his remarks on types and countertypes. Examples cited included Down's Syndrome (mongolism) with extra chromosome-21 material, in contrast to antimongolism with material missing; the *cri du chat* or deletion of the short arm of chromosome-5 syndrome in contrast to trisomy of the short arm of chromosome-5; and chromosome-18 trisomy versus 18-deletion syndrome. Lejeune pointed out that, in chromosomal imbalance, children may have all of their biochemical machinery at hand but that some of the reactions in vivo are running too fast or too slow. His concluding remarks were "This way of research must be investigated, for it is our only hope that someday we will be able to do something for those children, who, not having received an equitable patrimony, are, in the true sense of the term, the most disinherited of the children of man."

Irene Uchida (Winnipeg) presented the dermatoglyphic findings in chromosomal aberration syndromes, it being apparent that the strongest association exists between dermatoglyphics and the autosomal trisomy syndromes. Loss of part of the chromosome appears to have less effect on dermatoglyphic patterns than has extra chromosomal material.

J. A. F. Roberts (London) closed the 3-day meeting with a talk on "Reflections on twenty years' experience of genetic counseling." Roberts presented data regarding the attitudes of parents to genetic counseling advice which they had received. Approximately one-half of the couples given a good prognosis were, in fact, completely reassured. The other half were either doubtful, or did not believe the advice, or considered that even a very small risk was too big. People referred for genetic advice are, on the average, much above the general run of hospital patients in intelligence and in sense of responsibility. Although it is only a relatively small proportion of people who need genetic advice, those who need it need it badly.

Numerous others, expert in the various aspects of medical genetics, contributed to the meeting by participation in panel discussions pertinent to the role of human genetics in disease. There were approximately 350 attending the meeting, and proceedings of the meeting are being published.

The seminar was supported by a supplement to a training grant (Project 413) from Children's Bureau, HEW.

# Genetic Diagnosis in the Newborn

## A Part of Preventive Medicine

FREDERICK HECHT, M.D.*

EVERETT W. LOVRIEN, M.D.**

Genetics plays a major role in the practice of medicine. Genetics is to biology what atomic theory is to the physical sciences. The role of genetics in medicine is multifaceted.[5, 7] Our emphasis here will be on one facet: genetic diagnosis and counseling.

Some of the principles of genetic counseling follow:

1. Genetic counseling is an integral part of patient management.

2. The responsibility for genetic counseling rests with the physician caring for the patient. He should provide the counseling or make sure that it is done.

3. Genetic counseling must be based on an accurate diagnosis.

4. A family history in pedigree form should be obtained prior to counseling. Reported evidence of disease in relatives should be confirmed whenever this may affect the genetic counseling.

5. Health workers from other disciplines may need to be involved to help in diagnosis, counseling, and treatment of the patient and his family.

6. Genetic counseling does not include making decisions for the family. Certain decisions are the family's responsibility and right.

7. Genetic counseling involves concern for the emotional as well as the physical consequences of the disease in the family.

8. Genetic counseling should be initiated as early as possible after

Supported by a grant from the Children's Bureau for a genetics program and by U.S. Public Health Training Grant 1 To HD 00165 and Research Grant AM 13173.

the birth of a child in whom an hereditary disease is suspected. Once the pedigree has been obtained, the genetic diagnosis and counseling should be planned in stages.

## Family History Taking

No special knowledge is necessary for taking a genetic family history. Since the purpose of a pedigree is to present the family history visually, some uniformity in recording is necessary so that pedigrees from various sources can be read quickly and informatively. The index patient should be indicated first on the pedigree with an arrow. The patient's siblings are then recorded chronologically on the same line. All pregnancies, including miscarriages, abortions and stillbirths, are listed. Then the parents, their brothers and sisters, their children, and the grandparents are added to the pedigree. Husband and wife should be put at adjacent ends of their sibships, so that they can be connected by a line.

The family history generally comprises three generations. Each person's full name, date of birth and if deceased, date of death, should be recorded. Medical questions should be deferred until after the pedigree has been completed. This saves time, allows the family time to think about their relatives, and provides the opportunity for the historian to ask a logical series of questions.

Close relatives are generally most important, and certain minimal data should be recorded in every instance. These data include the ethnic origin, religious background, and birthplaces of the grandparents. One can diminish the risk of being offensive by commenting, "I am asking about ethnic origin because some diseases are more common in certain populations." Inquiry should be made as to whether there are any of the father's family names in the mother's family and vice versa. This leads to the question, "Are your families in any way related to each other?"

Religion is also noted. It is well known that some diseases are more prevalent in certain religious groups. Examples include pyruvate kinase deficiency and hair-cartilage hypoplasia in the Amish, and Tay-Sachs disease in Ashkenazic Jews. Knowledge of religious affiliation can also lead to church records such as the excellent genealogies kept by Mormons.

The place of residence of each household is indicated on the pedigree. This may be useful later in locating family members or in linking family groups. For example, we recently saw a family with polydactyly from a very small town in Oregon. While typing the patient's record, the secretary was alerted by the unusual name of the town. She looked through other pedigrees of patients with the same diagnosis and found another family from the same town. It could then be readily seen that these were branches of the same family.

The reliability of the informants must be assumed, but verification is often useful. Many times an older family member can provide information about a branch of the family that the younger members did not know existed. A family may bring records, bibles, and photographs of their family to provide additional verification of the pedigree and the diagnosis.

## Complete Medical History and Physical Examination

Appropriate physical examinations must be made in order to confirm the diagnosis and to counsel effectively. The index case and as many family members as possible should be examined when evaluating the pattern of inheritance.

Physical examinations also help define the severity of the disease. It is as important to inform the parents of a mongoloid child that their baby has heart disease as it is to inform them that trisomy 21 is usually sporadic. Parents want to know what medical complications to expect. Providing information which allows the family to plan ahead is part of genetic counseling.

Examination often rewards the careful observer in other ways. A family was being evaluated for Huntington's chorea and a careful medical student noted a small central starburst lens opacity in one of the children. Examination of other members of family revealed that congenital cataract was segregating as an autosomal dominant condition independently of Huntington's chorea.

Although patients seek genetic advice in regard to a particular genetic trait, they may have another condition which is also of importance. This may be overlooked unless an adequate family work-up is done. For example, a 19 year old pregnant woman was referred to the clinic by the obstetrical service. She was nearly 6 feet tall and had poor vision as a result of subluxated lenses. She was suspected of having homocystinuria. However, her urinary amino acids were normal. It was feared that she might have Marfan's syndrome and develop an aortic aneurysm during her pregnancy. However, her pregnancy went smoothly and her baby was normal. A pedigree and physical examination showed 34 cases of congenital cataract. Congenital cataracts, not Marfan's syndrome, were segregating in this family.

## Laboratory Studies

Reliable genetic counseling often depends upon accurate laboratory investigation. Few physicians would hesitate to order liver function tests for a jaundiced patient or an hematocrit or hemoglobin for an anemic patient. Similarly, it is necessary to utilize laboratory studies in addition to clinical data to evaluate certain genetic disorders. The desirability of laboratory tests should be determined *after* thorough appraisal of the pedigree and physical findings.

For example, chromosome studies may provide useful counseling information. The value of chromosome studies is typified by two siblings with mongolism plus diabetes. Each child had the usual features of mongolism, in which there are usually 47 chromosomes. However, these siblings had 46 chromosomes, and their mother and maternal grandfather had 45 chromosomes, including a D/21 translocation. The mother's brother was found to be carrying the same D/21 translocation. He recently asked about the risk of mongolism for his children because his wife was pregnant. We estimated a maximum risk of approximately 2 per cent. He and his wife now have the option of electing amniocentesis or awaiting the outcome of the pregnancy without further evaluation.

117

# GENETIC DIAGNOSIS

Genetic counseling depends upon three factors: an accurate family history; an exact diagnosis; and knowledge of the literature.

It is very important in counseling for the physician to be positive about the family history. In one family the oldest sibling of a child with maple syrup urine disease was found to be normal. Therefore the likelihood that this child was a carrier of maple syrup urine disease was 2/3. However, on blood grouping we found that the child's blood type was not compatible with that of her father. Later we learned that the mother knew this all along. The likelihood that the child really is a carrier of maple syrup urine disease is therefore 1/2. If parents possess information which qualifies an evaluation, counseling may be incorrect as well as ineffective.

Occasionally family studies lead to awkward situations and there may be reluctance in providing access to family records or in permitting family examinations. For example, when it was decided to draw blood on all members of a family for blood grouping, the mother revealed to the nurse that the first of her four children was not by her husband. She realized that nonpaternity would be detected and wanted the information to be kept from her husband. Her wish was respected.

Many genetic conditions require special investigations, and a proportion of cases may require a specialist's opinion. For example, in hemophilia it is important to distinguish hemophilia A, hemophilia B (Christmas disease or PTC deficiency) and Von Willebrand's disease. Hemophilia A and B are both X-linked recessive disorders; hemophilia B tends to be somewhat milder. Von Willebrand's disease is an autosomal dominant trait and is usually mild. The choice of treatment, the prognosis, and the genetic counseling for these three types of hemophilia are different. Amniocentesis for a woman who has a previous child with Von Willebrand's disease is valueless, since at present one can not diagnose this disorder prenatally; knowledge of the fetus's sex is not helpful since males and females both have a 50 per cent risk of being affected.

Genetic diseases need to be carefully distinguished from phenocopies which mimic them. For example, aniridia may be familial or sporadic. The familial type is inherited as an autosomal dominant trait with a 50 per cent risk of affecting the next born child. The sporadic form does not usually affect subsequent children, but it is associated with an increased risk of Wilms' tumor.

Unusual forms of a condition also need to be recognized since they may carry different risks of recurrence. For example, facial clefts, which are usually isolated anomalies with relatively low recurrence risks, may sometimes be part of a multiple congenital anomaly syndrome inherited as an autosomal dominant trait with a 50 per cent chance of recurrence.

Historically our knowledge of genetic disorders has evolved in a way which still influences our thinking about them.

X-LINKED DISEASES. Phenotypes resulting from mutant genes on the X chromosome present a characteristic pedigree pattern. They affect boys and their maternal uncles but skip their mothers. This pattern of transmission is so characteristic that the ancient Jewish Talmud stipulated that circumcision could be omitted for newborn males whose older brothers or maternal uncles were bleeders. A recent catalog of Mendelian phenotypes in man lists 10 per cent as X-linked.[6] By contrast the X chromosome represents only about 6 per cent of the length of the human haploid chromosome complement. The 68 traits on the human X chromosome constitute the largest number of gene loci known to be on a single mammalian chromosome. They include medically serious conditions such as hemophilia A and B, the Lesch-Nyhan syndrome, and one type of gout due to hypoxanthine-guanine-phosphoribosyl-transferase deficiency. Some X-linked disorders detectable in the newborn period are listed in Table 1.

AUTOSOMAL DOMINANT DISEASES. Traits in which large numbers of affected individuals occur in different generations are usually inherited as autosomal dominants. These disorders describe a vertical pattern on the pedigree. Some of these traits, such as polydactyly, have been known since the eighteenth century. Heritable congenital malformations and disorders with delayed onset of symptoms usually are dominants. The fundamental biochemical basis of most autosomal dominant conditions is still unknown. Table 2 lists some of these disorders which may be detected in newborn infants.

**Table 1.** *Some X-Linked Diseases Detectable in the Newborn**

Agammaglobulinemia, Swiss type
Albinism, ocular
Albinism-deafness syndrome
Aldrich's syndrome of thrombocytopenia, infection, and eczema
Angiokeratoma, diffuse: Fabry's disease
Cataract, congenital, total
Cataract, congenital, with microcornea
Deafness, congenital, perceptive type
Diabetes insipidus, nephrogenic
Ectodermal dysplasia, anhidrotic
Glucose-6-phosphate dehydrogenase deficiency
Granulomatous disease, chronic
Hemophilia A
Hemophilia B
Hydrocephalus due to aqueductal stenosis
Hypophosphatemic vitamin-D resistant rickets
Ichthyosis
Iris, hypoplasia of, with glaucoma
Lesch-Nyhan syndrome
Lowe's oculo-cerebro-renal syndrome
Megalocornea
Microphthalmia or anophthalmia with digital anomalies
Mucopolysaccharidosis type II: Hunter syndrome
Norris's disease: pseudoglioma
Ophthalmoplegia, external, and myopia
Retinoschisis
Van den Bosch syndrome: choroideremia, anhidrosis, skeletal deformity, and mental retardation

*References relating to each of the disorders listed are to be found in McKusick, V. A.: Mendelian Inheritance in Man. Baltimore, Johns Hopkins Press, 2nd ed., 1968.

**Table 2.** *Some Autosomal Dominant Diseases Detectable in the Newborn**

| | |
|---|---|
| Achondroplasia | Myotonia congenita: Thomsen's disease |
| Acrocephalosyndactyly: Apert's disease | Nail-patella syndrome |
| Angioneurotic edema, hereditary | Nemaline myopathy |
| Aniridia | Oculodentodigital dysplasia |
| Anonychia – ectrodactyly | Ophthalmomandibulomalic dysplasia |
| Antitrypsin deficiency | Ophthalmoplegia, familial static |
| Auriculo-osteodysplasia | Optic atrophy, congenital |
| Basal cell nevus syndrome | Osteogenesis imperfecta |
| Brachydactyly | Osteopetrosis: Albers-Schonberg disease |
| Camptodactyly | Osteopoikilosis |
| Cataract (some genetic forms) | Pachyonychia congenita |
| Cleft lip and/or palate with lip pits | Paramyotonia congenita of Eulenberg |
| Cleft lip and/or palate with popliteal web | Polydactyly |
| Cleidocraniodysostosis | Porphyria |
| Coproporphyria | Ptosis, hereditary |
| Crouzon's craniofacial dysostosis | Pupillary membrane, persistent |
| Deafness with ear pits | Radioulnar synostosis |
| Diabetes insipidus, neurohypophyseal type | Retinal aplasia |
| Dyschondrosteosis | Retinoblastoma |
| Ehlers-Danlos syndrome | Rieger's syndrome: dysgenesis of iris and |
| Elliptocytosis |    cornea, hypodantia (and myotonic |
| Epidermolysis bullosa with onychodystrophy |    dystrophy) |
| Hemoglobin, $\alpha$-chain mutants, e.g., Hb M | Spherocytosis, hereditary |
| Hemoglobin, $\gamma$-chain mutants | Split lower lip |
| Holt-Oram: heart-hand syndrome | Split-hand deformity: lobster-claw |
| Horner's syndrome |    deformity |
| Hyperbilirubinemia, Gilbert's type | Spondyloepiphyseal dysplasia, congenital |
| Joint laxity, familial | Supravalvular aortic stenosis |
| Kok's disease: hypertonia, exaggerated | Symphalangism |
|    startle reflex | Syndactyly |
| Leri's pleonosteosis | Triphalangeal thumb |
| Lymphedema, hereditary: Milroy's disease | Von Hippel-Lindau syndrome |
| Mandibulofacial dysostosis: Treacher Collins' | Von Willebrand's disease: pseudo- |
|    disease |    hemophilia |
| Marfan syndrome | Waardenburg's syndrome: white fore- |
| Moebius syndrome: congenital facial |    lock, heterochromia iridis, and |
|    paralysis |    deafness |
| Monilethrix | White sponge nevus of the mouth |

*References relating to each of the disorders listed are to be found in McKusick, V. A.: Mendelian Inheritance in Man. Baltimore, Johns Hopkins Press, 2nd ed., 1968.

AUTOSOMAL RECESSIVE DISEASES. Advances in medical biochemistry in the twentieth century have led to the recognition of a rapidly growing number of autosomal recessive phenotypes. The clinical recognition of these recessive conditions was slow because of the general pattern of outbreeding in man and the relatively small number of offspring born to any one couple. Autosomal recessive diseases, however, can be of major clinical importance. Examples are phenylketonuria, galactosemia, and maple syrup urine disease; in all of these control of diet is therapeutically helpful. The clinically normal heterozygote maintains the gene in the population in recessive disorders; generally, affected individuals of either sex are born of normal parents. The pedigree shows either a sporadic case or affected sibs, i.e., a horizontal pattern of inheritance. Some autosomal recessive conditions detectable in newborn infants are listed in Table 3.

CHROMOSOME DISEASES. Bartholin's syndrome (trisomy 13) and Down's syndrome (trisomy 21) were identified clinically in the seven-

## Table 3. *Some Autosomal Recessive Diseases Detectable in the Newborn**

Abdominal muscles, absence of, with
  urogenital malformation
Abetalipoproteinemia
Acatalasemia
Adrenal hyperplasia
Albinism
Alkaptonuria
Alpers' diffuse degeneration of cerebral gray
  matter
Amaurosis congenita of Leber I
Aminoacidurias
Amyotonia congenita
Analphalipoproteinemia: Tangier disease
Anemia, congenital hypoplastic
Anophthalmos, true or primary
Antitrypsin deficiency of plasma
Aplasia cutis congenita
Argininosuccinic aciduria
Arterial calcification, generalized, of infancy
Asphyxiating thoracic dystrophy of the
  newborn
Ataxia-telangiectasia
Atrichia with papular lesions
Behr's infantile hereditary optic atrophy
Bloom's syndrome: dwarfism with skin
  changes
Cataract, congenital or juvenile
Chondrodystrophia calcificans congenita
Citrullinuria
Cockayne's syndrome: dwarfism, marble
  epiphyses, etc.
Corneal dystrophy, band-shaped
Cretinism, athyreotic
Crigler-Najjar syndrome: nonhemolytic
  jaundice
Cystathioninuria
Cystic fibrosis of the pancreas
Cystinuria, types I, II, and III
Dandy-Walker syndrome
Deafmutism and functional heart disease
Deafmutism (some types)
Diastrophic dwarfism
Disaccharide intolerance
Ellis-Van Creveld syndrome
Epidermolysis bullosa, letalis
Factor X deficiency
Fanconi's pancytopenia
Fibrin-stabilizing factor deficiency
Fructose intolerance, hereditary

Galactosemia
Gangliosidosis, generalized
Gaucher's disease, type II
Glaucoma, congenital
Glutathione deficiency of erythrocytes
Glutathione reductase
Glycinemia
Glycogen storage disease, types I and II
Hallermann-Streiff syndrome
Heart-block, congenital
Hemivertebrae, multiple

Hemochromatosis, idiopathic neonatal, giant
  cell hepatitis
Hexokinase deficiency hemolytic anemia
Histidinemia
Holoprosencephaly, familial alobar
Homocystinuria
Hurler syndrome
Hyperglycinemia, isolated
Hyperlipoproteinemia, type I
Hyperlipoproteinemia, type V
Hyperlysinemia
Hyperprolinemia, types I and II
Hypoglycemia, leucine-induced
Hypophosphatasia
Hypoprothrombinemia
Hypotrichosis
Ichthyosiform erythroderma
Ichthyosis congenita
Isovalericacidemia
Krabbe's disease
Larsen's syndrome
Laurence-Moon-Biedl-Bardet syndrome
Leprechaunism
Lymphopenic hypergammaglobulinemia
Macular degeneration of the retina
Maple syrup urine disease
Marinesco-Sjögren syndrome
Morquio syndrome
Mesomelic dwarfism of the hypoplastic
  ulna, fibula and mandible type
Metatropic dwarfism
Methemoglobinemia
Microcephaly
Muscular atrophy, infantile
Nephrosis, congenital
Niemann-Pick disease
Oroticaciduria
Osteopetrosis
Phenylketonuria
Polycystic kidney, infantile, type I
Porphyria, congenital
PTA deficiency
Pycnodysostosis
Pyridoxine dependency
Pyruvate kinase deficiency
Reticulosis, familial histiocytic
Retinitis pigmentosa
Rothmund-Thomson syndrome
Sjögren-Larsson syndrome
Spastic diplegia, infantile type
Spastic paraplegia hereditary
Spongy degeneration of central
  nervous system
Suxamethonium sensitivity
Tay-Sachs disease
Thalassemias
Usher's syndrome
Weill-Marchesani syndrome
Wolman's disease
Xeroderma pigmentosum

*References relating to each of the disorders listed are to be found in McKusick, V. A.:
Mendelian Inheritance in Man. Baltimore, Johns Hopkins Press, 2nd ed., 1968.

121

teenth and nineteenth centuries, respectively. Only in the late 1950's and 1960's were they shown to be due to chromosome abnormalities. Human somatic chromosome methodology has in turn led to the discovery of new diseases such as Edward's syndrome (trisomy 18), the cri-du-chat syndrome (5p-syndrome), the 13q-syndrome, and so forth.

POLYGENIC DISEASES: SOME COMMON MALFORMATIONS.  Polygenic or multifactorial conditions are poorly understood. No adequate catalog of them, comparable to the invaluable compilation of Mendelian dominant, recessive, and X-linked traits in man,[6] is available. The gene loci in polygenic conditions have not been identified, nor is the number of loci known. However, a set of empiric risks of recurrence, some of which are listed in Table 1, are available. Some common malformations are polygenic (Table 4).

## GENETIC DISEASES IN THE NEWBORN PERIOD

Genetic diseases in the newborn period usually fall into two categories. One category represents "genetic emergencies." For example, a seriously ill child with the $D_1(13)$ trisomy syndrome may survive only a brief period of time. It is essential to examine the baby and obtain appropriate blood or skin samples to expedite cytogenetic studies. The other category of disorders is not medically urgent. For example, a child born with Turner's syndrome usually requires no emergency management, but does require adequate examination to document the diagnosis. Similarly, phenylketonuria is a genetic emergency; vitamin D-resistant rickets is not.

One recent innovation has greatly increased the need for genetic counseling. A public health screening program of all newborns, the Guthrie program, has been introduced into many communities. As a result, physicians caring for newborn infants in these communities are consulted by parents seeking advice for the interpretation of laboratory screening results and the management of their child.

Only a fraction of genetic diseases are detectable in the newborn infant. Some genetic diseases such as β-thalassemia never manifest themselves in the newborn period. Other genetic diseases, such as cystic fibrosis, are only partially expressed in the newborn period. A newborn infant with cystic fibrosis may have intestinal disease, but he may not have the pulmonary disease which so often develops in older children with cystic fibrosis. Further, to diagnose many genetic diseases in the newborn infant, the physician must know the family history. For example, the knowledge that an older sister had cystic fibrosis should prompt a sweat chloride test of the newborn baby. Similarly, knowledge that the father has emphysema due to antitrypsin deficiency may lead one to check the newborn's serum trypsin inhibitor capacity.

In the newborn period the baby and the mother are usually in the hospital. The father is also often nearby, assuring that at least two and often three generations of the family are available for study. An accurate family history, laboratory tests, or certain examinations by specialists can be done at this time that may be more difficult to obtain later. The

**Table 4.** *Counseling Figures for Some Common Malformations**

| | ANENCEPHALY OR MENINGO-MYELOCELE | CLEFT LIP PLUS OR MINUS CLEFT PALATE | CLEFT PALATE ALONE | PYLORIC STENOSIS | CONGENITAL DISLOCATION OF HIP | CLUBFOOT |
|---|---|---|---|---|---|---|
| Approximate incidence in general Caucasian population | 2/1,000 | 1/1,000 | 1/2,500 | 2/1,000 | 1/1,000 | 1/1,000 |
| Incidence in siblings of an affected child with unaffected parents | 3.4–4.8/100 | 4.9/100 | 2.0/100 | 3.2/100 (brothers 4.0 sisters 2.4) | 3.5/100 (brothers 0.5, sisters 6.3) | 2.8/100 |
| Incidence in children of an affected parent | | 4.3/100 | 6.0/100 | Affected father 4.6, Affected mother 16.2 | | 2.8/100 |
| References | 13, 15, 16 | 12, 17 | 11 | 10 | 17 | 9, 10 |

*Modified from Smith, D. W., and Aase, J. M.: Polygenic inheritance of certain common malformations. Evidence and empiric recurrence risk data. J. Pediat., 76:653, 1970. These data are applicable for these anomalies as isolated malformations, but not when they occur as a part of a multiple malformation syndrome.

parents of a child born with a serious genetic problem, such as a congenital malformation or a metabolic disorder, should receive prompt genetic counseling. The first affected child usually is a shock to the parents, for there is generally no suspicion before delivery. The birth of a second affected child is an even greater tragedy. Parents seek both recurrence risk figures and information about the medical consequences of the diagnosis.

## GENETIC COUNSELING

### Staging of Genetic Counseling

When a newborn child is thought to have a possible genetic disease the parents are anxious to know if the child is normal. However, the physician may need to counsel them in stages. This is illustrated by three cases from our experience:

CASE 1. *Down's syndrome*. A second child was born of a 25 year old woman. Her first child was normal. The newborn infant, however, was hypotonic, had a flat face with epicanthal folds, and single transverse (simian) palmar creases. These findings, plus the baby's general appearance (Gestalt) suggested to the physician who saw the baby in the nursery that the baby might have Down's syndrome. A colleague called in to examine the infant was similarly suspicious of Down's syndrome. They performed a dermatoglyphic study which showed high palmar axial triradii and arch tibial patterns on the soles of the feet; both of these are common findings in Down's syndrome. With this much information available the physician talked to the baby's parents and said something along these lines: "I do not know if the baby has Down's syndrome – mongolism – but I am concerned. I have just had Dr. Jones see the baby and he agreed with my concern. We could be mistaken. I hope we are because Down's syndrome usually results in retardation. I have asked for a chromosome study. We should have the results of this in about a week. I will be entirely honest with you. If the chromosome results show Down's syndrome I will tell you so. In any case, the baby is fine now and she can go home with you when you leave the hospital."

This provisional counseling was designed to give the parents adequate knowledge without undue delay. It was also aimed at letting the parents begin their readjustment promptly after the birth of the baby. The parents needed to be able to talk with the physician frequently in the days that followed.

The chromosome study did show trisomy 21 which is the most common type of chromosomal abnormality in Down's syndrome. The parents were seen again and told: "I am afraid the diagnosis was correct. The chromosome studies of your child do show an extra chromosome. I wish I had been wrong, but. . . . The outlook for your daughter is that she will probably be slow. Instead of walking at a year of age, like your older child, she will probably start walking somewhat later. We will test her periodically to see how she is doing so that you can plan for her education. No one can tell now to what extent she will be retarded. She is too young. We will work along with you on this. You are doing a good job with her. You are doing everything that can be done to benefit her. Incidentally, the cause of the extra chromosome is unknown. It is not due to any known event which happened to you or anything that you did."

The attempt here was to counsel in stages about the diagnosis, to relieve guilt, to provide support, and to set the stage for further counseling.

CASE 2. *Cleft palate*. A boy was born with a bilateral palate cleft. There was no cleft of the lip and the remainder of the physical examination was normal. The parents were shown the baby in the delivery room and told: "You have a fine normal boy. His palate did not close fully, but that can be done surgically." The baby's feeding was discussed with the parents and they practiced feeding him before taking him home from the hospital.

At an office visit a week to 10 days later the counseling was extended by a discussion of the pathogenesis of cleft palate. "The palate normally closes at about 60 days gestation; whatever happened occurred before that time. To the best of our knowledge cleft palate is *not* due to medicine you may have taken, accidents you had, thoughts you had, or anything you did." Then the presumed polygenic basis of cleft palate was discussed. The purpose of this discussion was not only to impart information but to relieve feelings of guilt as much as possible. The parents were given an appointment to the cleft lip and palate clinic where a multidisciplinary team worked with the baby and his parents to map out a program of treatment.

CASE 3. *Amniocentesis for prenatal diagnosis.* A couple had a child with Pompe's disease (glycogen storage disease type II due to α-glucosidase deficiency). They initiated another pregnancy and then belatedly learned of the possibility of prenatal diagnosis. They contacted our genetic counseling clinic and arranged for an amniocentesis. This was done. The α-glucosidase activity in amniotic fluid was normal and they were informed of the results. The amniotic cells were cultured for enzyme assays to provide confirmation of the results from the amniotic fluid. The parents will be counseled about these results as soon as they are available. When the baby is born, a sample of blood will also be taken for further confirmation. Again, the aim is to provide genetic data in stages as determined by the facts available at the time.*

## Presenting the Information

In order to provide parents with effective information so that they can arrive at a decision which they are qualified to make, the information must be clearly stated. For example, quoting specific risk figures to a couple may be confusing if they are told the risk is 5 per cent to a subsequent offspring. The same couple may understand better when they are told the risk of having an affected child is 1 in 20. The use of specialized nomenclature, such as "heterozygote," "segregation," etc., should be avoided.

Genetic counseling requires at least as much listening as talking. For example, we saw a young man and his wife for counseling. She had a petit mal seizure disorder and was taking anticonvulsants. Her first pregnancy resulted in a premature infant son with a tracheo-esophageal fistula, who expired shortly after birth. Her second child was a male who was normal at birth but became cyanotic a few hours later and died. Autopsy revealed transposition of the great vessels. The pedigree was interesting in that the mother was one of 17 siblings, eight of whom died in the early neonatal period with either prematurity or congenital malformations. One had anencephaly. We wrote to the various attending physicians, hospitals, and relatives to obtain autopsy reports, medical records, and family records. The wife was evaluated in our clinic by a neurologist. Cytogenetic studies indicated that the parents were chromosomally normal. The couple was told that we could not recognize a common pattern to the malformations suggesting a genetically deter-

---

*As the case actually developed (after completion of this manuscript), amniotic cell cultures had no detectable enzymatic activity. This led the parents to elect a therapeutic abortion, which yielded a fetus with no detectable α-glucosidase activity in liver, muscle, or other tissues—i.e., with Pompe's disease.

mined syndrome. Similarly, we could not find evidence to indicate that anticonvulsants produce multiple congenital malformations in the offspring when taken by expectant mothers. We concluded that we did not regard them as a high risk couple, but that we might be wrong.

The couple subsequently had a miscarriage, and about a year later a child who died at birth with a nonpatent trachea, cleft palate, ambiguous genitalia, six fingers on one hand and four on the other, club feet, deformed ears and imperforate anus. The delivery room nurse and the obstetrician obtained cord blood for chromosome analysis. Cytogenetic evaluation revealed a normal male chromosome complement.

The couple again requested genetic counseling. Their obstetrician had advocated tubal ligation. A careful reappraisal of the entire situation was held. The couple finally stated that they had a conviction that they had not previously revealed to us. They felt that their case was different from that of other couples with congenitally malformed offspring since none of their defective children had lived. The children had not been a great burden to them. They both felt a strong need to have children. Even if we told them that their risk was high, for example as high as 50 per cent, they would elect to accept that risk. Thus, they planned to have another pregnancy. Meanwhile, they did do one new thing; they began adoption proceedings so that they could begin to raise a family.*

**Useful Advice to Be Given**

Genetic risks tend to separate themselves into two groups: those in which the risk is worse than 1 in 10; and those which are better than 1 in 20. There are few in between. Complications arise from alternative modes of inheritance. Every complication of the genetic scheme reduces the proportion of affected persons among relatives. As the genetics become more obscure the empirical chances of having an unaffected child improve. Simple uncomplicated transmission usually means moderate to high risk; puzzling pedigrees are usually coupled with a more hopeful outlook.

It is not part of the task of counseling to advise patients whether or not they should have children. An explanation of the chances of having an affected offspring is what is required so that the parents can make up their own minds. Parents are generally relieved when the facts about risk are given. Unsophisticated people should not be underestimated; they often have clear insight into the meaning of the odds.

The chance that any pregnancy will result in a serious malformation or mental retardation is about 2 to 3 per cent. Therefore the parents need to be told that their genetic risks must be added to the usual background risk for everyone of 2 to 3 per cent. Different people have different

---

*Since the completion of this paper, two similar mothers have been described. They were receiving trimethadione or paramethadione for the control of seizures and had a total of nine pregnancies, all of which ended either in spontaneous abortion or in the birth of an abnormal child. When the drugs were withdrawn, all three subsequent pregnancies ended with the birth of a normal child. (German et al., Lancet, 2:261, 1970.)

thresholds for acceptable risks. Some people will accept a risk of 1 in 4. Others 1 in 20. Some will not accept a risk of 1 in 100.

No one can be given an absolute guarantee. Complete reassurance is unwise; a risk, though minimal, may still be present.

### Future of Genetic Counseling in the Newborn Period

The future need for genetic counseling will greatly increase for everyone caring for newborn infants. As a result of improved prenatal care and obstetrical service, the proportion of infant care devoted to "crisis treatment" is diminishing. At the same time, the care of the chronically handicapped child is becoming more important. The next few years may see an increased interest in the detection of late onset genetic disorders before they are manifest. Genetic disorders which are manifest in early adulthood have until recently been of little concern to the pediatrician. Traditionally, such disorders as coronary artery disease, chronic obstructive emphysema, and acute intermittent porphyria have been designated as belonging to the province of the internist. With the development of screening tests which can be used to identify individuals at risk, pediatricians will need to identify newborn infants who have a high probability of developing a genetic disorder later as young adults. The infants will need to be followed in an attempt to establish effective therapy. For example, newborn infants who are born into a family with coronary disease should have lipoprotein analysis while they are still in the hospital. The same is true for $\alpha_1$-antitrypsin determination in families with emphysema and porphobilinogen in families with porphyria.

Dr. Richard Sleeter has made the statement that we should no longer think of "present illness" in our traditional pediatric evaluations, but rather think "family history." If we think "family history," utilize effective laboratory and screening methods, and are familiar with the literature, genetic counseling moves rapidly from the category of a medical luxury to the position of a pediatric necessity.

### Individuals Qualified to Provide Genetic Counseling

J. A. Fraser Roberts makes the point, "Giving genetics advice to patients is one particular aspect of medical practice, and, just as with any other, must be accepted as an art, though an art founded on scientific principles." From our experience we believe that any qualified member of the health team can provide genetic counseling. This includes family doctors, pediatricians, internists, obstetricians, other medical specialists, speech pathologists, audiologists, clinical psychologists, and other qualified health professionals. The person providing genetic counseling must know the relevant facts. Cases which are not understood should be referred for further diagnostic study and counseling. The general principles of genetic counseling should also be observed by whoever is providing the counseling.

### Genetic Counseling in Practice

Several physicians who are in practice have participated in a training period in our genetics clinic. We have asked them for their views on

127

genetic counseling in practice.* Some of the points they made are as follows:

1. Most families do not initiate discussion of genetic problems. The discussion may need to be opened by the physician.

2. Adolescents are often interested in discussing genetic diseases in their family and may wish to receive genetic counseling.

3. The premarital examination is an appropriate time for a genetic history and counseling by physicians in general or obstetrical practice.

4. There is danger in practice of having a one-time counseling session from which the patients may take only a portion of the counseling. Therefore, genetic counseling should be planned in somewhat the same way as the treatment of school problems. At least half-hour appointments should be scheduled at a time when interruptions are least likely to occur. Also, a minimum of one follow-up visit should be scheduled in order to answer additional questions and to reiterate the facts.

5. One should collaborate with other members of the health team, as needed, including obstetricians, clinical psychologists, orthopedists, etc.

6. Genetic counseling is challenging and rewarding work for a physician in practice.

## REFERENCES

KEY SOURCES OF INFORMATION FOR GENETIC COUNSELING

1. Gardner, L. I., ed.: Endocrine and Genetic Diseases of Childhood. Philadelphia, W. B. Saunders, 1969.
2. Gellis, S. S., and Feingold, M.: Atlas of Mental Retardation Syndromes. Visual Diagnosis of Facies and Physical Findings. U.S. Government, Printing Office, Washington, D.C. 20402.
3. Gorlin, R. J., and Pindberg, J. J.: Syndromes of the Head and Neck. New York, McGraw-Hill Book Co., 1964.
4. International Directory of Genetics Services, compiled by Henry T. Lynch. May be obtained free-of-charge on request from the National Foundation, Professional Education Department, 800 Second Avenue, New York, New York 10017.
5. McKusick, V. A.: Human Genetics. Englewood, New Jersey, Prentice-Hall, Inc., 2nd ed., 1969.
6. McKusick, V. A.: Mendelian Inheritance in Man. Catalog of Autosomal Dominant, Autosomal Recessive and X-Linked Phenotypes. Baltimore, Johns Hopkins Press, 2nd ed., 1968.
7. Roberts, J. A. F.: An Introduction to Medical Genetics. New York, Oxford University Press, 5th ed., 1970.
8. Stanbury, J. B., Wyngaarden, J. B., and Fredrickson, D. S., eds.: The Metabolic Basis of Inherited Disease. New York, McGraw-Hill Book Co., 2nd ed., 1966.

REFERENCES TO RECURRENCE RISKS FOR MALFORMATIONS

9. Böök, J. A.: A contribution to the genetics of congenital clubfoot. Hereditas, 34:289, 1948.
10. Carter, C. O.: The inheritance of common congenital malformations. Progr. Med. Genet., 4:59, 1965.
11. Curtis, E. J., Fraser, F. C., and Warburton, D.: Congenital cleft lip and palate. Amer. J. Dis. Child., 102:853, 1961.

---

*We thank Drs. Raymond Corwin (Portland), Ronald Stuart (Medford), and James Strain (Denver) for these ideas.

12. Fogh-Andersen, P.: Inheritance of cleft lip and cleft palate. Copenhagen, Ejnar Munks-gaard Forlag, 1942.
13. MacMahon, B., Pugh, T. F., and Ingalls, T. H.: Anencephalus, spina bifida and hydro-cephalus. Incidence related to sex, age, race, and season of birth and incidence in siblings. Brit. J. Prev. Soc. Med., 7:211, 1953.
14. Record, R. G., and Edwards, J. H.: Environmental influences related to the aetiology of congenital hip disease. Brit. J. Prev. Soc. Med., 12:8, 1958.
15. Record, R. G., and McKeown, T.: Congenital malformations of the central nervous system. III. Risk of malformations in sibs of malformed individuals. Brit. J. Soc. Med., 4:217, 1950.
16. Williamson, E. M.: Incidence and family aggregation of major congenital malformations of central nervous system. J. Med. Genet., 2:161, 1965.
17. Woolf, C. M., Woolf, R. M., and Broadbent, T. R.: A genetic study of cleft lip and palate in Utah. Amer. J. Human Genet., 15:209, 1963.

# Counselling in Diseases Produced Either by Autosomal or X-Linked Recessive Mutations[1]

O. Frota-Pessoa[2], J. M. Opitz[3], J. G. Leroy and K. Patau

A number of inherited diseases, in spite of apparent phenotypic homogeneity, are due to the homozygous state of an autosomal recessive mutation in some pedigrees and an X-linked recessive mutation in others. At times it is possible to distinguish the two types on clinical, physiological or biochemical grounds; but in practice genetic counseling with respect to such diseases must often be given when the pattern of inheritance is doubtful. This paper presents a method for estimating the risk of being affected for a child born to a *normal female* having one or more brothers affected by this type of disease. The method is applied to the mucopolysaccharidoses (syndromes of Hurler and Hunter).

## 1. Different Kinds of Risk

Let us consider a sibship born to normal parents and composed of $N$ individuals, among which $n$ are normal, $i$ being normal females and $(n-i)$ normal males, and $(s>1)$ are affected, $j$ being affected females

[1] Paper No. 1175 from the Genetics Laboratory, University of Wisconsin, Madison.

[2] Supported at the University of São Paulo by Rockefeller Foundation Research Grant 63060/28 and at the University of Wisconsin by US Department of State Research Grant 64-030-A and by NIH Grant GM 08217.

[3] Supported by Grants from the National Foundation and NIH Grants GM 08217 and 15422-01.

and *(s-j)* affected males. What is the probability $P$ for a child born to one of the normal females by a normal husband to be affected? We assume that the woman in question has no previous children (by this or other marriages) and that the same applies to all of her sibs, or at least, that pertinent information regarding the phenotypes of all other relatives is lacking. If the mutation responsible for the disease is autosomal, $P$ assumes the value

$$p = \frac{2}{3} \cdot c \cdot \frac{1}{4} = \frac{c}{6} \tag{1}$$

where $c$ is the probability of the child's father being a heterozygous carrier of the autosomal recessive gene. On the other hand, if the disease in the pedigree is produced by an X-linked gene, $P$ becomes $p'$ and

$$p' = \frac{1}{2} \cdot \frac{1}{4} = \frac{1}{8} \tag{2}$$

It is seen that, barring father–daugther incest, $p'$ is always greater than $p$: about three times greater if the child's parents are first cousins ($c \simeq \frac{1}{4}$) and about 38 times greater if they are not consanguineous and the frequency of the autosomal gene in the population is 0.01 (and at equilibrium $c \simeq 0.02$).

A third possibility is that the propositus is a sporadic case and his or her condition results from a fresh mutation. This is improbable in the case of the autosomal type of the disease, but the frequency of male propositi owing their condition to fresh mutation in the X-linked locus is not negligible, especially when the disease is severe or lethal. The probability $p''$ that a sister of a fresh mutation case has an affected child is small (although considerably greater than the mutation rate in the population, see PATAU and NACHTSHEIM, 1946) and will be considered negligible here.

These differences in risk according to the genetic nature of the disease show the importance, for counselling, of estimating the probabilities $w$, $w'$ and $w''$ that the affection of a given propositus is due, respectively, to the transmission of the autosomal gene, to the transmission of the X-linked gene, or to fresh mutation in an X-linked locus. We assume, as a sufficiently good approximation, that these are mutually exclusive possibilities, so that $w + w' + w'' = 1$. If, for instance, the value of $w$ approaches unity the sibship can be considered to belong to the autosomal type and counselling must be given on this basis. On the other hand, if the three probabilities have significant values, the probability $P$ must be calculated as the weighted mean of $p$, $p'$ and $p''$, the weights being $w$, $w'$ and $w''$ respectively. Making $p'' = 0$:

$$P = wp + w'p' \tag{3}$$

Let us consider now the probability $P_m$ for a child of one of the *normal males* in the sibship to be affected. The value corresponding to $p$ is then the same as in equation 1 but $p'$ may be taken as zero since a normal male could not be a carrier of the sex-linked gene producing the disease. As a result, equation 3 reduces to:

$$P_m = wp \tag{4}$$

Consider now a sample of independent sibships drawn randomly from the population by ascertainment through affected children (truncate selection) including only sibships born to normal parents. Two sibships in the same pedigree will be both included in the sample only if ascertained independently through different propositi. Let $r$, $r'$ and $r''$ be the prior probabilities ($r+r'+r''=1$) of a random sibship in this sample having its propositus affected as a consequence, respectively, of the transmission of an autosomal gene, of the transmission of an X-linked gene and of a fresh mutation in an X-linked locus. Methods for evaluating these prior probabilities will be presented below. The values of $r$, $r'$ and $r''$ are the best estimates of $w$, $w'$ and $w''$, respectively, in the absence of all information about the structure of the sibship. As soon as the number and the sex of the sibs or even the sex of the propositus alone are ascertained, these probabilities have to be combined with the partial probabilities contributed by the new information for an evaluation of the overall probabilities $w$, $w'$ and $w''$. For instance, if the sibship includes more than one affected individual, $w''$ becomes zero since, in practice, only sporadic cases will be considered as derived from fresh mutation. On the other hand, if the sibship includes one or more affected females, both $w$ and $w''$ become zero and we know for sure that the inheritance is autosomal. Of course, in the last case no probabilistic computation is called for; but in the first case, although being sure that the sibship in question belongs to the transmission category, we have still to compute the probabilities of the sibship being of the autosomal and of the X-linked type respectively. Finally, if the propositus in the sibship in question is a sporadic case, then the three possibilities remain open and we must compute $w$, $w'$ and $w''$.

If a sample of sibships approaching the characteristics described above is available, estimates of $r$ can be reached by two methods. The first method does not depend on $r''$ and leads to estimates of $r$ and $(1-r) = (r'+r'')$. The second method discriminates the three probabilities and is more efficient than the first method, since it uses more information. However, the determination of $r''$ demands a previous evaluation of $r$ (by means of the first method).

## 2. First Estimate of the Prior Probabilities

Let $d$ be the number of sibships in the sample with one or more affected females but no affected male; $e$ the number of sibships including both male and female affected sibs; $D$ the total number of sibships in the sample; and $r_1$ the estimate of $r$ obtained by this method. The $(d+e)$ sibships containing affected females are obviously of the antosomal type; besides, assuming that the disease is not sex-influenced, $d$ more sibships of the autosomal type containing one or more affected males but no affected female are expected to be included in the sample of sibships. Therefore

$$r_1 = \frac{2d + e}{D} \quad \text{and} \tag{5}$$

$$1 - r_1 = \frac{D - 2d - e}{D} \tag{6}$$

A variant of this method consists in considering only the propositus of all sibships in the sample and taking twice the number of females among them, divided by $D$, as an estimate of $r$. This is preferable when data on the rest of the sibs is scarce, suspected to be very inaccurate or biased.

Estimation of $r'$ must be postponed until $r''$ has been estimated.

## 3. Estimation of the Frequency of the Fresh Mutation Cases

Let $a_m$ and $a_f$ be the observed number of affected males and affected females, respectively, and $a = a_m + a_f$ be the total number of affected individuals in the sample of sibships. The proportion $a_m/a$ of males

133

among the affected individuals is expected to be $\frac{1}{2}$ in the autosomal and 1 in the X-linked fraction of sibships. In all sibships taken together $a_m/a$ is expected to be the weighted mean of these values. Using as weights $r$ and $(1-r)$

$$\frac{a_m}{a} = \frac{1}{2} r + (1-r) = \frac{2-r}{2} \tag{7}$$

Hence, the fraction $a'$ of affected males owing their disease to the X-linked gene is

$$a' = \frac{1-r}{(2-r)/2} = \frac{2(1-r)}{2-r} \tag{8}$$

Among these $a'$ X-linked cases, a fraction $a''$ owe their condition to fresh mutations. For X-linked recessive detrimentals the mutation rate, at equilibrium, is $\mu = (1-f) x/3$, where $f$ is the fitness of affected males and $x$ is their frequency at birth [HALDANE, 1935]. From this it is concluded that $(1-f)/3$ of the total number of males affected by the X-linked type of the disease must be fresh mutation cases. Therefore

$$a' = \frac{(1-f)a'}{3} = \frac{2(1-r)(1-f)}{3(2-r)} \tag{9}$$

Since there are $a_m$ affected males in the sample of sibships, the number of individuals in the sample who are fresh mutation cases is

$$a''a_m = \frac{2a_m(1-r)(1-f)}{3(2-r)} \tag{10}$$

Each individual affected as a result of fresh mutation is the only affected member of his sibship; therefore the number of sibships belonging to the fresh mutation category is also $a''a_m = r''D$ and their frequency in the sample of sibships is

$$r'' = \frac{a''a_m}{D} = \frac{2a_m(1-r)(1-f)}{3D(2-r)} \tag{11}$$

Using the estimate $r_1$ (expression 5) for $r$ in expression 11, the value of $r''$ is determined. This done, an estimate $r'_1$ of $r'$ can be reached by subtracting $r''$ from $(1-r_1)$ in expression 6.


## 4. Second Estimate of the Prior Probabilities

Each of the sibships belonging to the fresh mutation category contains just one affected individual (the male propositus). In this they differ from the transmission group of sibships which have, in the sample, an average number $\bar{s}$ of affected individuals per sibship greater than one. Taking this into account, the total number $a$ of affected individuals in the sample of sibships can be expressed as

$$a = (\bar{s}r + \bar{s}r' + r'')\,D \qquad (12)$$

The number $a_m$ of affected males is

$$a_m = \frac{1}{2}\,\bar{s}r + \bar{s}r' + r'')\,D \qquad (13)$$

The frequency of males (sex-ratio) among the affected individuals is

$$\frac{a_m}{a} = \frac{\dfrac{1}{2}\bar{s}r + \bar{s}r' + r''}{\bar{s}r + \bar{s}r' + r''} \qquad (14)$$

The value of $\bar{s}$ is

$$\bar{s} = \frac{a - r''D}{D - r''D} \qquad (15)$$

After substituting in expression 14 the value in 15 for $\bar{s}$ and the value $(1-r-r'')$ for $r'$ (and remembering that $a-a_m = a_f$) we arrive at

$$r = \frac{2a_f(1 - r'')}{a - Dr''} \qquad (16)$$

Applying to 16 the estimate of $r''$ given in expression 11, our second estimate, $r_2$, of $r$ can be computed. A corresponding second estimate, $r'_2$, of $r'$ is given by

$$r'_2 = 1 - r_2 - r'' \qquad (17)$$

## 5. Probabilities Depending on the Structure of the Sibship

For reaching estimates of $w$, $w'$ and $w''$ the prior probabilities $r$, $r'$ and $r''$ have to be combined to the partial probabilities associated to the composition of the sibship in question.

Since the sibship contains obligatorily at least one affected individual (the propositus) the probability is $\frac{1}{2}$, 1 and 1 for, respectively, the case of autosomal gene, transmission of the X-linked gene and fresh X-linked mutation. The probabilities associated with the individuals in the sibship besides the propositus are shown in table I.

We can write now the probabilities $q$, $q'$ and $q''$ of a sibship of $N$ individuals including at least one affected (the propositus) being composed of $i$ normal females, $(n-i)$ normal males, $j$ affected females and $(s-j)$ affected males under the hypotheses of, respectively, auto-

135

*Table I.* Probabilities of the different types of sibs (propositus excluded) for the three possible types of sibships

| Types of sibships | normal female | normal male | affected female | affected male |
|---|---|---|---|---|
| Autosomal gene | 3/8 | 3/8 | 1/8 | 1/8 |
| Transmission of sex-linked gene | 1/2 | 1/4 | 0 | 1/4 |
| Mutation of sex-linked gene | 1/2 | 1/2 | 0 | 0 |

somal transmission, X-linked transmission and X-linked mutation. Since we are interested in the probability of a precise sequence of individuals, we omit the customary combinatorial factor in the expressions below

$$q = \frac{1}{2} \left( \frac{3}{8} \right)^n \left( \frac{1}{8} \right)^{s-1} \tag{18}$$

$$q' = \left( \frac{1}{2} \right)^i \left( \frac{1}{4} \right)^{n-i} \left( \frac{1}{4} \right)^{s-1} \tag{19}$$

$$q'' = \left( \frac{1}{2} \right)^n \tag{20}$$

It is understood that $(s-j) > 1$ nulls $q''$ and $j > 0$ nulls both $q'$ and $q''$.

## 6. *The Overall Probabilities*

Normalizing the products $rq$, $r'q'$ and $r''q''$, probabilities $w$, $w'$ and $w''$ are obtained

$$w = \frac{rq}{rq + r'q' + r''q''} \tag{21}$$

$$w' = \frac{r'q'}{rq + r'q' + r''q''} \tag{22}$$

$$w'' = \frac{r''q''}{rq + r'q' + r''q''} \tag{23}$$

If the sibship under study is of the sporadic type with male propositus ($j=0$; $s=1$), expressions 18 and 19 become simpler and expressions 21 to 23 can be written as follows

$$w = \frac{3^n r}{3^n r + 2^{n+i+1} r' + 2^{2n+1} r''} \tag{24}$$

$$w' = \frac{2^{n+i+1} r'}{3^n r + 2^{n+i+1} r' + 2^{2n+1} r''} \tag{25}$$

$$w'' = \frac{2^{2n+1} r''}{3^n r + 2^{n+i+1} r' + 2^{2n+1} r''} \tag{26}$$

For sibships with more than one affected male and no affected female ($j=0$; $s>1$), $q''$ (and $w''$) becomes zero and expressions 24 and 25 reduce to

$$w = \frac{3^n r}{3^n r + 2^{n+i+1} r'} \tag{27}$$

$$w' = \frac{2^{n+i+1} r'}{3^n r + 2^{n+i+1} r'} \tag{28}$$

Computations of $w$ and $w'$ according to formulae 24 and 25 or 27 and 28 are made taking into account expressions 16 and 17 for the values of $r$ and $r'$. Once $w$ and $w'$ are found, the risks $P$ and $P_m$ are calculated according to formulae 3 and 4. For purely counseling purposes $w''$ need not to be computed because, $p''$ being considered as zero, formulae 3 and 4 do not contain $w''$.

### 7. Case of Benign Diseases or Defects

Formula 11 shows how $w''$ depends on $f$, the fitness of the affected males. For lethal diseases ($f=0$), $r''$ is not negligible, but it can be considered so for diseases or defects which are not severe and do not impair obviously the average number of children produced by the affected males. In those cases the risks expressed in formulae 3 and 4 can be estimated in a simpler way.

Because $r''$ is considered as zero, $r+r' = 1$ and the value given by formula 6 becomes an estimate, $r'_1$, of $r'$.

The second estimate of $r$ and $r'$, presented in section 4, becomes more direct. Formulae 14 and 16 reduce respectively to

$$\frac{a_m}{a} = \frac{\frac{1}{2}r + r'}{r + r'} = \frac{2-r}{2} \qquad \text{and} \qquad (29)$$

$$r = \frac{2a_f}{a} \qquad (30)$$

The value of $r$ in expression 30 is the second estimate $r_2$ of $r$. Also $r'_2$ (expression 17), becomes simply $1-r_2$.

The simplification brought about by $r''$ being negligible makes the use of a third method for evaluating $r$ practical and allows the combination of it with the second method discussed above for obtaining a more efficient estimate of the prior probabilities.

## 8. Third Estimate of the Prior Probabilities

Let $b_m$ and $b_f$ be the observed numbers of normal males and normal females, respectively, and $b = b_m + b_f$ the total number of normal individuals in the sample of sibships. The frequency $b_m/b$ of males (sex-ratio) among the normal individuals is expected to be $\frac{1}{2}$ in the autosomal fraction and $1/_3$ in the X-linked fraction of sibships. In all sibships

$$\frac{b_m}{b} = \frac{1}{2}r + \frac{1}{3}(1-r) = \frac{2+r}{6} \qquad \text{and} \qquad (31)$$

$$\frac{b_f}{b} = \frac{4-r}{6} \qquad (32)$$

Expression 32 leads to the following estimates, $r_3$, of $r$ and, $r'_3$, of $r'$

$$r_3 = 4 - \frac{6b_f}{b} \qquad (33)$$

$$r'_3 = \frac{6b_f}{b} - 3 \qquad (34)$$

## 9. Second and Third Estimates of r and r' Combined

The second estimate, $r_2$, of $r$ (expression 30) is more efficient than the third ($r_3$, expression 33) because the expected value of $a_f/a$ varies from zero to one while $b_f/b$ varies only from $\frac{1}{2}$ to $\frac{2}{3}$ when one goes from exclusively autosomal sibships to exclusively X-liked ones.

138

Also $r_2$ tends to be more accurate than $r_3$ because the sex of affected individuals is in general verified by the researcher studying them, but the sex of their normal sibs is often obtained through information. This makes it advisable to use $r_2$ and $r'_2$ alone when the data have been collected routinely by persons not aware of the importance of recording accurately the sex of the propositi's sibs. However, when the data are adequate, it is more appropriate to use the information from the sex-ratio of both the affected and the normals and reach a combined estimate $r_4$ of $r$ (and $r'_4$ of $r'$) by the maximum likelihood method.

The expected frequencies of the observed numbers $a_m$, $a_f$, $b_m$ and $b_f$ are respectively $(2-r)/2$ (expression 29), $r/2$, $(2+r)/6$ (expression 31) and $(4-r)/6$ (expression 32). Their combined probability is

$$P_o = \frac{a!}{a_m!a_f!}\left(\frac{2-r}{2}\right)^{a_m}\left(\frac{r}{2}\right)^{a_f}\frac{b!}{b_m!b_f!}\left(\frac{2+r}{6}\right)^{b_m}\left(\frac{4-r}{6}\right)^{b_f} \qquad (35)$$

$$P_o = (2-r)^{a_m}\ r^{a_f}\ (2+r)^{b_m}\ (4-r)^{b_f}\ \frac{a!b!}{a_m!a_f!b_m!b_f!}\left(\frac{1}{2}\right)^{a}\left(\frac{1}{6}\right)^{b} \qquad (36)$$

From this the value of $r$ which maximizes $P_o$ is found in the usual manner:

$$L = \log P_o = a_m\log(2-r) + a_f\log r + b_m\log(2+r) + b_f\log(4-r) + K$$

$$\frac{dL}{dr} = -\frac{a_m}{a-r} + \frac{a_f}{r} + \frac{b_m}{2+r} - \frac{b_f}{4-r} = 0$$

$$-(8r + 2r^2 - r^3)a_m + (16 - 4r - 4r^2 + r^3)a_f + (8r - 6r^2 + r^3)b_m - (4r - r^3)b_f = 0$$

$$(a + b)r^3 - 2(a + a_f + 3b_m)r^2 - 4(a + a_m - 2b_m + b_f)r + 16a_f = 0 \qquad (37)$$

The value of $r$ satisfying 37 is the maximum likelihood estimate, $r_4$, of $r$. Once it is found, the estimate $r'_4 = 1 - r_4$ is obtained.

### 10. Application to the Mucopolysaccharidoses

Human mucopolysaccharidoses include at least one X-linked form (Hunter's syndrome) and four autosomal forms (Hurler's syndrome, I-cell disease- LEROY et al., 1968-, San Filippo and Scheie forms). Differential diagnosis can now be made by the specialist on clinical grounds and on the basis of anamnestic data [LEROY et al., 1966]. Data from the revision by JERVIS [1950] and a newer sample of 49 sibships collected and studied by LEROY et al. [1966] are analysed in table II.

*Table II.* Analysis of two samples of sibships [JERVIS, 1950, and LEROY *et al.*, 1966], each sibship containing a propositus affected by mucopolysaccharidosis

| Classes of sibships and individuals | Numbers included in samples | |
|---|---|---|
| | JERVIS | LEROY *et al.* |
| A. Sibships with only females among the affected sibs $(d)$[1] | 32 | 13 |
| B. Sibships with both males and females among the affected sibs $(e)$ | 11 | 1 |
| C. Sibships with only males among the affected sibs | 67 | 35 |
| D. Total number of sibships in the sample $(D)$ | 110 | 49 |
| I. Affected males $(a_m)$ | 93 | 42 |
| II. Affected females $(a_f)$ | 52 | 15 |
| III. Normal males $(b_m)$ | – | 27 |
| IV. Normal females $(b_f)$ | – | 53 |
| V. Normal, sex unknown | – | 3 |
| VI. Miscarriage, sex unknown | – | 17 |
| VII. Miscarriage, female | – | 1 |

[1] Symbols between parentheses have the same meaning as in the text formulae.

Classes V and VI in table II were disregarded in the estimation of $r$, $r'$ and $r''$ since zygotes of unknown sex do not contribute relevant information for this purpose. The female miscarriage in Class VII was assumed to be not affected. Its inclusion as an affected female would alter only slightly the results. Table III presents the estimates of the prior probabilities according to the methods discussed in this paper and, for sake of comparison, according to purely clinical criteria $(r_{c1})$, for the sample of LEROY *et al.* (33 autosomal sibships among 49).

## 11. Examples

Having evaluated the prior probabilities for the mucopolysaccharidoses (table III) we may consider now some representative sibships among those included in LEROY *et al.* sample. Table IV describes the composition of these sibships and presents the results of computations leading to the evaluation of the overall probabilities related to them.

*Table III.* Estimation of the prior probabilities for mucopolysaccharidoses based on the sibship samples analysed

| Parameters | JERVIS | LEROY et al. |
|---|---|---|
| $r_{c1}$ (clinical estimation) | – | 0.673 |
| $r_1$ (formula 5) | 0.682 | 0.551 |
| $r_2$ (formula 16) | 0.691 | 0.511 |
| $r'_1 = 1 - r_1 - r''$ | 0.184 | 0.272 |
| $r'_2$ (formula 17) | 0.175 | 0.312 |
| $r''$ (formula 11) | 0.134 | 0.177 |

*Table IV.* Probabilities for a child of a normal member ($P$ for female, $P_m$ for male) of the specified sibships (selected from LEROY et al. sample) to be affected by mucopolysaccharidosis (the values $r = 0.511$, $r' = 0.312$, $r'' = 0.177$ were used; see table III)

| Sibship | Children born alive $(N)$[1] | | | | Prior probabilities[2] | | | Overall risks[3] | |
|---|---|---|---|---|---|---|---|---|---|
| | Affected $(s)$ | | Normal $(n)$ | | | | | | |
| | Male | Female | Male | Female | | | | | |
| | $(s-j)$ | $(j)$ | $(n-i)$ | $(i)$ | w | w' | w'' | P | $P_m$ |
| Chipman | 0 | 1 | 0 | 0 | 1.000 | 0 | 0 | (0.003) | (0.003) |
| Fagan | 1 | 0 | 0 | 0 | 0.343 | 0.419 | 0,238 | (0.053) | (0.001) |
| Gonsalves | 1 | 0 | 2 | 0 | 0.360 | 0.196 | 0.444 | (0.026) | 0.001 |
| Wright | 1 | 0 | 2 | 1 | 0.297 | 0.215 | 0.488 | 0.028 | 0.001 |
| Coutts | 1 | 0 | 2 | 2 | 0.241 | 0.232 | 0.527 | 0.029 | 0.001 |
| Hawm | 1 | 0 | 0 | 4 | 0.142 | 0.548 | 0.311 | 0.070 | (<0.001) |
| Brian | 1 | 0 | 1 | 5 | 0.120 | 0.412 | 0.468 | 0.052 | <0.001 |
| Arnan | 1 | 0 | 2 | 4 | 0.105 | 0.181 | 0.410 | 0.023 | <0.001 |
| Honesberg | 2 | 0 | 0 | 0 | 0.291 | 0.709 | 0 | (0.090) | (0.001) |
| Greene | 3 | 0 | 1 | 1 | 0.200 | 0.800 | 0 | 0.101 | 0.001 |

[1] Symbols as defined in the text.

[2] According to formulae 24 to 26 except sibships 9 and 10 for which formulae 18 to 23 were used.

[3] According to formulae 3 and 4 and assuming no consanguinity and $c = 0.02$.

( ) These figures are given even though the sibship contains no individuals to whom they apply.

## Summary

The estimate of risks in the case of diseases which can be due either to autosomal or to X-linked recessive genes becomes dubious when the affected individuals in the pedigree are few and all are males. This paper develops a method for calculating such risks combining probabilities derived from (a) the incidence of the two forms of the disease in the population, (b) the estimated frequency of fresh mutations and (c) the structure of the sibship under study. The method is applied to the mucopolysaccharidoses.

## Acknowledgements

We are indebted to Dr. J. F. CROW for his interest in the development of this paper. We are particularly grateful to Dr. C. C. COTTERMAN for his critical review of this paper and his many helpful comments and suggestions.

## References

1. HALDANE, J. B. S.: The rate of spontaneous mutations of a human gene. J. Genet. *31:* 317–326 (1935).
2. JERVIS, G. A.: Gargoylism (Lipochondrodystrophy): A study of 10 cases with emphasis on one formes frustes of the disease. Arch. Neurol. Psychiat. *63:* 681–712 (1950).
3. LEROY, J. G. and CROCKER, A. C.: Clinical definition of the Hurler-Hunter phenotypes. Amer. J. Dis. Child *112:* 518–530 (1966).
4. LEROY, J. G. and CROCKER, A. C.: Studies on the genetics of the Hurler-Hunter syndrome. In: Inborn errors of sphingolipid metabolism (Pergamon Press, Oxford 1966).
5. LEROY, J. G.; OPITZ, J. M. and DEMARS, R.: I cell disease: a newly recognized, recessively inherited disorder, resembling Hurler's disease. In preparation.
6. PATAU, K. and NACHTSHEIM, H.: Mutations- und Selektionsdruck beim Pelger-Gen des Menschen. Z. Naturforsch. *1:* 345–348 (1946).

# Prenatal Genetic Diagnosis

# Culture of cells obtained by amniocentesis

CARLO VALENTI and TEHILA KEHATY

A tissue culture technique has been described which, if applied to fetal cells obtained by amniocentesis, has yielded successful cell growth in 20 of 24 cases. Amniotic fluid volumes greater than 30 ml. were associated with the greatest rate of success. Satisfactory chromosome preparations were obtained in 17 cases, the failures being due to bacterial contamination. The technique represents a valuable diagnostic tool for effective genetic counseling and for the study of early human development.

Fetal cells obtained by amniocentesis, cultivated in vitro, and subjected to cytogenetic and biochemical analysis can mirror the genetic make-up of the unborn fetus. When done early in pregnancy this procedure offers an effective method for genetic counseling for selected high-risk persons, such as carriers of chromosomal translocations. It may also be indicated for the discovery of trisomies suspected in older patients or in mothers who already have affected offspring. Although several investigators have succeeded in culturing fetal cells prenatally, only two descriptions of the techniques employed have appeared in the literature. Steele and Breg[1] reported cell growth in 12 of 62 cultures, with karyotyping in only two of these. Jacobson and Barter[2] have achieved success in 62 of 92 cultures. Since neither method yielded satisfactory results in this laboratory, amniocentesis was used, as reported here, by which success was achieved in 83 per cent of the cases.

## Method

The placenta is located by an ultrasound technique, which can be used as early as the fourteenth week of pregnancy.[3] With aseptic conditions and local anesthesia, a 20 gauge 5 inch spinal needle with stylet is inserted through the abdominal wall, preferably on the midline, but always away from the placental site. After the stylet is removed, the amniotic fluid (AF) is withdrawn slowly into a plastic syringe. The AF is centrifuged at 42× g for 5 minutes and the supernate discarded. The cell pellet is resuspended in 1.5 ml. of fetal calf

144

serum (Hyland Laboratories) and placed in a 60 by 15 mm. plastic Petri dish. No cell viability count is deemed necessary. A No. 1, 43 by 50 mm. cover glass, trimmed to fit the Petri dish, is placed over the cells and the dish is stored at 37° C. for one hour. Eagle medium (3.5 ml.) with a concentration of aminoacids and vitamins, two and four times greater than usual,[4] respectively, is added. The Petri dish is then placed in an atmosphere of 8 per cent $CO_2$. The culture medium is changed on the third or fourth day, and approximately once a week thereafter. Occasionally after 2 weeks, and usually after 4 weeks, a monolayer of clear, fusiform, fibroblast-like cells, showing at least 3 per cent mitotic figures, will be noted. The culture is then split by inverting and transferring the cover glass to another Petri dish. Enough elements are adherent to the cover glass to assure their survival. Both cultures are refed. The cells on the cover glass are maintained as cell line, with a weekly 1:2 split subcultivation rate. The cells in the original container are exposed to Colcemide (0.006 per cent) for 4 hours and dislodged by trypsin (0.25 per cent). They are then suspended in warm hypotonic saline solution (0.95 per cent sodium citrate) for 15 minutes, spread on slides, air-dried, and stained with acetic orcein, with the same technique adopted for chromosome preparations from peripheral blood cultures.[5]

## Results

Twenty-four amniocenteses were performed in 22 patients (Table I). One patient, a balanced carrier of D/G chromosome translocation, was subjected to amniocentesis three times; the first cell culture failed (No. 9). The amniocentesis was repeated 2 weeks later; this cell culture (No. 11) provided the cytogenetic diagnosis of D/G translocation Down's syndrome in the unborn fetus. During the subsequent interruption of the pregnancy by intra-amniotic instillation of hypertonic saline solution, a third AF sample was obtained from which cells were successfully cultivated (No. 16). This case has been reported elsewhere.[6] Case No. 23 was a 37-year-old pregnant woman, who was concerned about her risk of bearing a Mongoloid baby. In two other instances the patients requested the analysis of fetal cells for fear of cytogenetic effects by LSD which had been ingested during the first trimester. Case No. 24 is a patient affected by severe hyperemesis gravidarum, who had been treated with barbiturates and chlorpromazine throughout 28 weeks of amenorrhea. Amniocentesis was performed in 7 cases of Rh immunization and 8 of therapeutic abortion. In two additional cases the AF was obtained during cesarean sections at term.

Cell growth was obtained in 20 out of 24 attempts (83 per cent). There were 17 satisfactory chromosome preparations (71 per cent). Except for Case Nos. 11 and 16, no numerical nor significant structural chromosomal aberrations were observed.

Because of bacterial contamination poor chromosome preparations were obtained in Case Nos. 6 and 12. Although cell growth was satisfactory for cytogenetic study, the Case No. 1 cells were fixed and stained for morphological studies.

The four failures of cell growth occurred when amniocentesis was performed at 15 and 36 weeks of amenorrhea (Nos. 3 and 7), at 10 weeks in No. 9 (a patient in whom a second amniocentesis provided good cell cultures), and at term (No. 17).

In four cases, Nos. 1, 2, 3, and 4, the AF was mailed to the laboratory and had been in transit for 1 to 4 days. Three of the 4 samples were successfully cultured.

The AF volume varied from 8 to 165 ml. All the failures occurred when the

*Table I.* Cultures of fetal cells obtained by amniocentesis

| Case No. | Duration of amenorrhea (weeks) | Clinical condition | Volume of amnioic fluid (ml.) | Cell growth | Chromosome preparations | |
|---|---|---|---|---|---|---|
| | | | | | Time lapse from amniocentesis (days) | Quality |
| 1 | 22 | Rh immunization | 10 | + | * | * |
| 2 | 22 | Rh immunization | 10 | + | 32 | Satisfactory |
| 3 | 15 | Rh immunization | 14 | - | — | — |
| 4 | 24 | Rh immunization | 10 | + | 29 | Satisfactory |
| 5 | 12 | Therapeutic abortion, medical | 30 | + | 21 | Satisfactory |
| 6 | 24 | Ingestion of LSD | 20 | + | 11 | Poor to satisfactory |
| 7 | 36 | Rh immunization | 20 | - | — | — |
| 8 | 25 | Rh immunization | 15 | + | 25 | Satisfactory |
| 9† | 16 | t D/G carrier | 28 | - | — | — |
| 10 | 14 | Therapeutic abortion, rubella | 40 | + | 34 | Satisfactory |
| 11† | 18 | t D/G carrier | 46 | + | 22 | Satisfactory |
| 12 | 16 | Therapeutic abortion, psychiatric | 22 | + | 32 | Poor |
| 13 | 8 | Therapeutic abortion, rubella | 20 | + | 20 | Satisfactory |
| 14 | 14 | Therapeutic abortion, psychiatric | 85 | + | 21 | Satisfactory |
| 15 | 12 | Therapeutic abortion, rape | | | | |
| 16† | 23 | t D/G carrier | 24 | + | 33 | Satisfactory |
| 17 | 40 | Cesarean section | 165 | + | 32 | Satisfactory |
| 18 | 35 | Rh immunization | 8 | - | — | — |
| 19 | 24 | Therapeutic abortion, rubella | 9 | + | 30 | Satisfactory |
| | | | 48 | + | 14 | Satisfactory |
| 20 | 18 | Therapeutic abortion, rubella | 15 | + | 30 | Satisfactory |
| 21 | 40 | Cesarean section | 65 | + | 25 | Satisfactory |
| 22 | 22 | Ingestion of LSD | 47 | + | 21 | Satisfactory |
| 23 | 15 | Advanced maternal age | 39 | + | 29 | Satisfactory |
| 24 | 28 | Hyperemesis gravidarum | 48 | + | 24 | Satisfactory |

*The cell cultures, actively growing, were fixed and stained for morphological studies.
†Amniocentesis performed in the same patient.

volume was less than 30 ml. The time interval between amniocentesis and chromosome preparations ranged from 14 to 42 days, averaging 26.6 days.

### Discussion

The fetal and maternal risks involved in amniocenteses are small.[7] Between the fourteenth and the seventeenth week of gestation, the placenta and the fetus can be readily identified by the ultrasound technique, a harmless procedure[8] which allows selection of a safe site for the transabdominal insertion of the needle. No complications were noted in the present series.

The sources of the cells obtained by amniocentesis are multiple, and they include epithelia such as those lining the amnion, the genitourinary, alimentary and respiratory tracts, and the skin.[9] The karyopicnotic squamous cells that make up the majority of the elements suspended in the AF are not viable, never adhered to the glass and were eliminated at the first medium change. The few viable cells which contribute to the establishment of the cultures may have originated from the respiratory tract.[2] The cells in all cultures looked like fibroblasts—never epithelioid. The use of a stylet and the avoidance of the placental site reduce the risk of maternal cell contamination to a remote possibility.

Neither the duration of amenorrhea nor the clinical conditions seem to explain the failures of cell growth. Of three amniocenteses performed in one case at intervals of 2 and 5 weeks during the second trimester, two succeeded and one failed. All four failures occurred when the AF volume was less than 30 ml. A larger series could lend greater reliability to this figure.

Bacterial contamination was probably responsible for the two cases of poor, unusable chromosome preparations. Although blood in the AF made microscopic monitoring of the cells difficult, there was no interference with cell growth in the three cases in which this occurred (Nos. 13, 15, and 20).

It is conceivable that amniocentesis may become a valuable diagnostic tool in detecting fetal chromosomal and cytological damage due to irradiation, viral infections, and teratogenic drugs. The cytological study of the unborn fetus may allow salvage of normal babies, previously doomed by adverse statistical evaluations. Furthermore, the diagnosis of inherited metabolic disorders may be possible by assaying the cells for enzymatic activity. It seems reasonable to expect success in Niemann-Pick and Gaucher diseases, homocystinuria, cystathionuria, and glycogen storage diseases.[10] The timing of the amniocentesis between the fourteenth and seventeenth week of amenorrhea will allow for chromosome preparations when interruption of pregnancy if indicated can still be induced with relative safety.

**REFERENCES**

1. Steele, M. W., and Breg, W. R.: Chromosome analysis of human amniotic-fluid cells, Lancet 1: 383, 1966.
2. Jacobson, C. B., and Barter, R. H.: Intrauterine diagnosis and management of genetic defects, Am. J. Obst. & Gynec. 99: 796, 1967.
3. Gottesfeld, K. R., Thompson, H. E., Holmes, J. H., and Taylor, E. S.: Ultrasonic placentography—a new method for placental localization, Am. J. Obst. & Gynec. 96: 538, 1966.
4. Eagle, H.: Aminoacids metabolism in mammalian cell cultures, Science 130: 432, 1959.
5. Valenti, C., and Vethamany, S. K.: Functional anatomy of a cytogenetic service, Am. J. Obst. & Gynec. 99: 434, 1967.
6. Valenti, C., Schutta, E. J., and Kehaty, T.: Prenatal diagnosis of Down's syndrome, Lancet 2: 220, 1968.
7. Creasman, W. T., Lawrence, R. A., and Thiede, H. A.: Fetal complications of amnio centesis, J. A. M. A. 204: 949, 1968.
8. Smyth, M. G.: Animal toxicity studies with ultrasounds at diagnostic power levels, in Grossman, C. C., Holmes, J. H., Joyner, C., and Purnell, E. D., editors: Diagnostic ultrasound, New York, 1966, Plenum Press, Inc., p. 296.
9. Austin, C. R.: Sex chromatin in embryonic and fetal tissue, Acta cytol. 6: 61, 1962.
10. Uhlendorf, B., and Nadler, H. L.: Personal communication.

# Prenatal detection of genetic defects

Henry L. Nadler, M.D.

DURING THE PAST DECADE, the development of a number of procedures has made possible the prenatal detection and management of certain genetic defects, especially those referred to as inborn errors of metabolism[1] and the abnormalities of chromosomes.

Programs have been instituted for the detection of genetic disorders in the neonatal period[2, 3] with the hope that early diagnosis and therapy might significantly modify the natural history of the disease. In galactosemia,[4] maple syrup urine disease,[5] and adrenogenital syndrome,[6] early diagnosis and treatment may be life-saving. In other conditions, such as phenylketonuria,[7] early diagnosis and treatment may be responsible for decreasing the degree of mental deficiency. Excellent reviews of hereditary metabolic disorders have been published by Stanbury and associates,[8] Hsia,[9] and Harris.[10]

Tremendous growth has occurred in the field of cytogenetics since Tjio and Levan[11] conclusively established the human chromo-

*Supported by Grants Nos. 5 RO1 HD 02752 and TI AM 5186 from the National Institutes of Health, Public Health Service.*

some diploid number of 46. Lejeune and associates,[12] in 1959, proved the chromosomal basis of Down's syndrome. One year later, other investigators[13, 14] documented the familial transmission of a chromosomal aberration in two families with Down's syndrome. These findings were followed by the definition of a number of congenital malformation syndromes associated with specific chromosomal aberrations. Since adequate treatment or correction of these disorders has not been available, emphasis has been placed on prevention in the forms of genetic counseling and/or therapeutic abortion.

Many approaches are possible for the treatment and prevention of genetic defects (Table I), but early diagnosis is necessary for all. This paper will review the work on the prenatal detection of genetic defects. The detection of Rh iso-immunization has been recently reviewed,[15-17] and only the data pertaining to the risks of transabdominal amniocentesis will be discussed.

### AMNIOCENTESIS

Amniocentesis has been used as a diagnostic aid since the early 1930's.[14] There has been widespread acceptance and utilization of this procedure since the demonstration of its place in the management of Rh iso-immunization.[19-21] The technique of transabdominal amniocentesis has been reasonably standardized and is summarized by Freda[16] and Queenan.[22] The procedures described by these authors are those used in obtaining amniotic fluid after the middle of the second trimester of pregnancy.

Well over 8,000 transabdominal amniocenteses have been performed with minimal maternal and fetal morbidity or mortality.[16-23] Burnett and Anderson[23] reviewed the hazards of amniocentesis and were able to find only two cases of maternal mortality, and 13 cases of maternal morbidity; the lat-

149

**Table I.** Approaches to the treatment and prevention of hereditary metabolic disorders[8]

| Approach | Disorder and treatment |
|---|---|
| Supply missing protein | Agammaglobulinemia: γ-globulin administration |
| Limit intake of precursor which may undergo toxic accumulation | Galactosemia: removal of galactose from diet |
| Supply missing metabolites | Orotic aciduria: feed cytodylic and uridylic acids |
| Environmental manipulation | Primaquine sensitivity: avoidance of drugs known to include hemolysis |
| Depletion of stored substances | Wilson's disease: penicillamine and BAL |
| Use of metabolic inhibitors | Gout: allopurinol |
| Limit "undesirable" genes | Genetic counseling and/or abortion |
| Genetic engineering | None as yet |

ter included amnionitis, maternal hemorrhage, abdominal pain, and peritonitis. No cases of perforation of the bladder or bowel have been reported. The fetal mortality appears to be greater than the maternal; fetal deaths due to abruptio placenta, amnionitis, and fetal hemorrhage[23-25] have been reported. Puncture of the fetus has been reported in seven cases.[25-27] The possibility for disruption of the fetomaternal circulation and consequent iso-immunization is a controversial question. Some investigators have demonstrated rapidly rising antibody titers following amniocentesis for Rh iso-immunization,[28-29] but controlled studies have failed to establish any relationship between the two.[30, 31] It should be pointed out that these results were obtained in studies of transabdominal amniocentesis performed primarily in the third trimester of pregnancy, and any generalization as to the risks in earlier stages of pregnancy are not justified.

Transabdominal amniocentesis has been performed from 8 to 20 weeks of pregnancy in over 200 cases,[32-36] in the vast majority immediately prior to the interruption of pregnancy. No maternal complications were observed, and in over 50 pregnancies carried to term, neither infant morbidity nor mortality has been reported. Some risk to the fetus has been demonstrated when amniotic fluid is obtained by vaginal amniocentesis.[32]

On the basis of the anatomic, physiologic, and developmental changes of the fetus and mother during the first half of pregnancy, as well as the experience gained in performing transabdominal amniocentesis during this period, the most suitable time to perform this procedure in the early stages of pregnancy would appear to be at 16 weeks of fetal gestation. Fig. 1 illustrates the relative size of uterus, amniotic sac, amniotic fluid, and baby at 8, 12, and 16 weeks of pregnancy.

## AMNIOTIC FLUID

Wagner and Fuchs[37] measured amniotic fluid volumes in seven patients at 12 weeks of pregnancy and found a range of 8 to 85 ml. The volume of amniotic fluid measured at 17 weeks of pregnancy ranged from 166 to 574 ml. with a mean of 225 ml. Plentl[38] states that at 10 weeks of pregnancy the average volume of amniotic fluid is 30 ml. and it gradually increases to 350 ml. at 20 weeks. The subjects of amniotic fluid volumes, measurements, and circulation have been reviewed by Plentl[38] and Jacoby.[39]

**Supernate.** Amniotic fluid is composed of 98 to 99 per cent water with 1 to 2 per cent solids. The inorganic constituents of am-

151

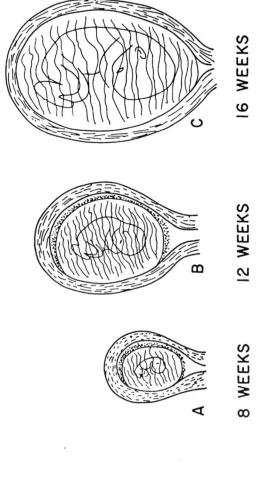

A          B          C

**8 WEEKS     12 WEEKS     16 WEEKS**

**Fig.** 1. Schematic illustration of the relative size of uterus, amniotic sac, and the fetus at 8, 12, and 16 weeks of pregnancy.

niotic fluid are quite similar to extracellular fluid, and the solids are equally divided between organic solids and proteins. An excellent review of the composition of amniotic fluid including its proteins, has recently been published.[40] Some investigators claim that the proteins are of maternal origin,[41, 42] while others[43, 44] present evidence attempting to show their fetal origin. The relative amounts of amnio acids in amniotic fluid have been studied[40] and appear to be similar to the concentration of amino acids in maternal plasma. A number of enzymes and hormones have been found in amniotic fluid.[40]

Jeffcoate and associates[45] and Fuchs[46] have been able to establish the diagnosis of the adrenogenital syndrome in utero by measuring the levels of 17-ketosteroids and pregnanetriol in amniotic fluid obtained during the thirty-ninth week of pregnancy. Fuchs[46] has also examined amniotic fluid from a mother who had previously borne a child with cystathionuria; no abnormalities were found in the amniotic fluid, and a normal infant was born.

Graven[47] has shown that samples of amniotic fluid obtained during the latter half of pregnancy have significant levels of lecithin, phosphatidylmono and phosphatidyldimethyl ethanolamines, and phosphatidic acid, presumably of fetal pulmonary origin. Graven and associates[48] have proposed a genetically determined "RDS predisposition factor" which, when present, predisposes a mother to deliver low–birth-weight infants who develop the respiratory distress syndrome. Graven[47] reported the absence of lecithin and phosphatidyl ethanolamines and a reduction of phosphatidic acid in the amniotic fluid of a mother in labor at 34 weeks of gestation. This infant developed severe respiratory distress, as had her previous children and those of her sister. This finding, if corroborated, may allow for early

153

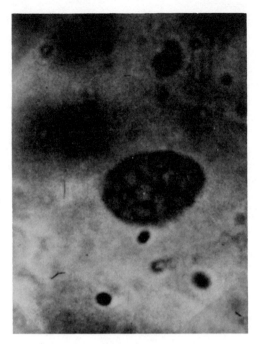

**Fig. 2.** Amniotic fluid cell demonstrating a sex chromatin mass at the periphery of the nucleus.

detection and management of babies likely to develop the respiratory distress syndrome. It is quite possible that many other disorders may be diagnosed in utero if techniques become available to measure abnormal metabolites and small increments or decreases of substances normally present at different stages of fetal gestation.

**Desquamated amniotic fluid cells.** The utilization of the cellular material found in amniotic fluid, which has been shown to be derived from amnion and fetus,[49] initially focused upon the technique of sex chromatin analysis for the antenatal determination of sex.[50-58] Fig. 2 illustrates a sex chromatin mass in the nucleus of an amniotic fluid cell. The presence of sex chromatin in amniotic fluid cells has been useful for the management of pregnancies in women heterozygous for X-linked recessive disorders such as hemophilia and muscular dystrophy.[59, 60] It should be emphasized that prenatal sex determination does not establish the diagnosis of an X-linked recessive disorder but merely yields more information upon which to base the management of such a pregnancy. The intrauterine detection of two X-linked recessive disorders, glucose-6-phosphate dehydrogenase deficiency and X-linked uric aciduria, will be discussed in the section on cultivated amniotic fluid cells.

Fuchs and associates[61] and others[62, 63] have been able to demonstrate immunogenetic markers in desquamated amniotic fluid cells. The ability to determine the ABO blood group of the fetus may prove valuable in the detection of genetic disorders which are linked to the ABO blood group locus. Gordon and Brosens[64] have reported a direct relationship between fetal age and the ability of these desquamated cells to stain orange with nile blue sulfate. This may be of value in the management of pregnancy in which the maturity of the fetus is unknown.

**Cultivation of amniotic fluid cells.** Recently, a number of investigators have demonstrated the ability to culture amniotic fluid cells.[32, 65-68] At the present time, 34 of 44 samples have been successfully cultivated in our laboratory, including 17 of 19 obtained prior to 20 weeks of gestation. Successful cultivation is defined as the ability to maintain the culture after two subcultures. The procedure involves collection of 2 to 10 c.c. of amniotic fluid by transabdominal amniocentesis. After approximately 18 to 25 days in cultures, the cells are trypsinized and subcultured. Three to five days later the cells are subcultured a second time and can now be used for cytogenetic and biochemical analysis. (Fig. 3 illustrates the appearance of the cells in culture at 0, 10, and 28 days.)

155

An important variable in the ability to cultivate amniotic fluid cells appears to be an as yet unidentified substance found in fetal calf serum. One lot of fetal calf serum differs from another in its ability to stimulate the growth of fetal cells. In two of three instances in which human fetal albumin was used in place of fetal calf serum, the time from planting the culture to subculture was reduced by 70 per cent, allowing the cells to be utilized for specific tests much more rapidly.

The ability to successfully cultivate amniotic fluid cells is related to the stage of pregnancy at which the sample is obtained. In general, the earlier in pregnancy the sample is obtained, the greater the likelihood of successful cultivation. Dancis[69] studied material from women with Rh iso-immunization obtained during the last trimester of pregnancy and, with the vital dye, eosin Y, was able to demonstrate that only 25 to 50 per cent of the cells were viable. In our experience using trypan-blue, the total number of viable cells increases with increasing gestational age while the percentage of viable cells decreases from a high of 50 to 70 per cent in the early stages of pregnancy to a low of 20 to 45 per cent during the last trimester. Steele and Breg,[65] using trypan-blue, reported finding fewer viable cells at earlier gestational stages.

**Chromosome studies.** Steele and Breg[65] reported successful chromosome analysis in **2 of 12 cases** in which cultures grew. In addition, they refer to a personal communication in which Klinger reports culturing amniotic fluid cells with a normal male karyotype. Thiede and associates[66] obtained satisfactory metaphase spreads in 3 of 11 cultures in which definite growth was demonstrated. Two were 46, XY, and one was 46, XX. In each case the sex as predicted by chromosome analysis corresponded to the

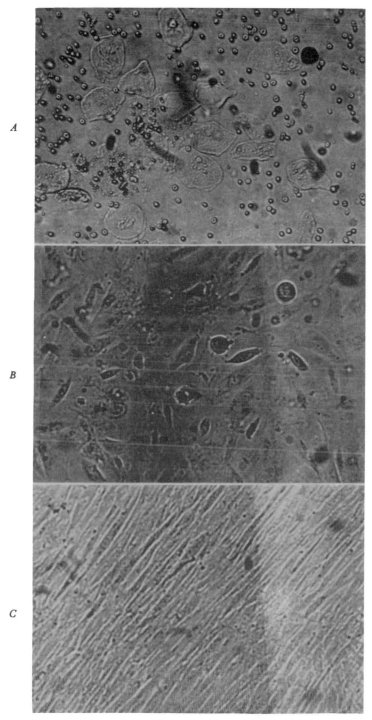

**Fig. 3.** Appearance of amniotic fluid cells in culture at *A,* 0 days, *B,* 10 days, and *C,* 28 days.

phenotypic sex of the infant. Jacobson and Barter[32] have reported the largest series of cultured amniotic fluid cells in which cytogenetic studies have been performed. Successful cultures, defined as producing satisfactory karyotypes, were obtained in 57 of 85 cases. A diagnostic amniocentesis was done in three cases of genetic high-risk pregnancies. In one case, A-18, amniocentesis was performed at 17 weeks of pregnancy in a 22-year-old D/D translocation carrier. Chromosome analysis using the cultivated cells demonstrated that the fetus was a D/D translocation carrier. Postnatal studies confirmed the intrauterine studies. In Case A-21, transabdominal amniocentesis was performed at 18 weeks of gestation in a known D/G translocation carrier. Cultivated cells were shown to have a normal 46, XX, chromosomal complement and a normal female was delivered at term. In Case A-38, amniocentesis was performed at 26 weeks on a woman who had previously delivered an infant with trisomic Down's syndrome. A normal 46, XX, karyotype was obtained which was confirmed with the birth of a normal female.

Nadler[34] reported successful cultivation of amniotic fluid cells in 27 of 37 cases. The sex of the fetus was determined by chromosome analysis using cultivated amniotic fluid cells, and in every instance the predicted sex was confirmed after delivery by examination of the external genitalia or after therapeutic abortion by chromosome analysis of the cultured abortion material. Amniocentesis has been performed during three pregnancies of mothers known to have D/G translocation. In one case the procedure was performed prior to a scheduled therapeutic abortion, and in the remaining two it was utilized as an aid in the management of the pregnancy. In Case I,[34] cultivated amniotic fluid cells, obtained by amniocentesis performed on a carrier of a D/G translocation prior to scheduled abortion at 10 weeks of pregnancy, demonstrated the presence of cells with a karyotype consistent with a male with a translocation form of mongolism (46, XY, t D/G, 21+). This finding, was confirmed utilizing the abortion material. In Case II,[34] amniotic fluid was obtained at 10 weeks of pregnancy from a known carrier of a D/G translocation. Chromosome analysis using cultivated amniotic fluid cells revealed the presence of 46 chromosomes, XX, normal karyotype. A repeat amniocentesis at 16 weeks again demonstrated a normal karyotype. A normal female with a normal chromosomal complement was delivered at term. In Case III, chromosome analysis using cultivated amniotic fluid cells obtained by amniocentesis at 16 weeks of pregnancy from a carrier of a D/G translocation revealed the presence of 46 chromosomes, XX, including the D/G translocation. On the basis of this finding a therapeutic abortion was performed at 20 weeks of fetal gestation and chromosome analysis of the cultured abortion material confirmed the chromosomal finding as being consistent with the diagnosis of Down's syndrome.

**Biochemical studies.** Biochemical studies of cultivated amniotic fluid cells have been reported by Nadler,[67] Uhlendorf and coworkers,[68] and Dancis.[69] The enzymes listed have been demonstrated in cultivated amniotic fluid cells obtained as early as 10 weeks of fetal gestation:

Acid phosphatase[67]
Alkaline phosphatase[67]
$\alpha$-glucosidase[67]
$\alpha$-keto-isocaproate decarboxylase[68, 71]
$\beta$-glucuronidase[67]
Cystathionine synthase[68]
Galactose-1-phosphate uridyl transferase[67]
Glucocerebrosidase[68]
Glucose-6-phosphate dehydrogenase[67]

Hypoxanthine-guanine phosphoribosyl transferase[68, 72]

Lactate dehydrogenase[67]

Phytanic acid $\alpha$-hydroxylase[68]

6-phosphogluconic dehydrogenase[67]

Sphingomyelinase[68]

Valine transaminase[69]

The intracellular distribution of glucose-6-phosphate dehydrogenase, lactate dehydrogenase, acid phosphatase, $\alpha$-glucosidase, and $\beta$-glucuronidase in cultivated amniotic fluid cells at all stages of fetal gestation have been shown to be similar to their distribution in fibroblasts derived from skin biopsies of children and adults.[74] Quantitative differences in glucose-6-phosphate dehydrogenase activity at diffrent stages of fetal gestation have been reported.[67] Glucose-6-phosphate dehydrogenase activity in cultivated amniotic fluid cells obtained after the sixteenth week of pregnancy is similar in males and females. The glucose-6-phosphate dehydrogenase activity in cells derived from two female fetuses decreased during the next six weeks both in vivo and in vitro. Simultaneous analysis of sex chromatin revealed 8 to 12 per cent positive cells in cultures derived from the two female fetuses at 10 weeks, as compared with the usual range of 25 to 35 per cent found in cells derived from female fetuses after 16 weeks of gestation. After six weeks in culture the percentage of sex chromatin positive cells had increased to 28 per cent. An elevated glucose-6-phosphate dehydrogenase activity associated with a lower than normal percentage of sex chromatin positive cells in these two female fetuses, followed by a change to normal levels, suggest that inactivation of an X-chromosome might be taking place both in vivo and in vitro.

Studies utilizing starch-gel electrophoresis have demonstrated qualitative differences of glucose-6-phosphate dehydrogenase and lactate dehydrogenase, while failing to demon-

Table II. Familial metabolic disorders demonstrable in tissue culture

| Disorder | Deficient enzyme or mutant phenotype |
|---|---|
| Acatalasemia[78] | Catalase |
| Branched-chain ketonuria[79] (maple syrup urine disease) | Branched-chain α-keto-isocaproate decarboxylase*[71, 80] |
| Chediak-Higashi syndrome[81] | Cytoplasmic inclusions |
| Citrullinemia[82] | Argininosuccinate synthetase |
| Cystathionuria[83] | Cystathionase*[83] |
| Cystic fibrosis[84] | Metachromatic granules |
| Cystinosis[85] | Increased free-cystine |
| Galactosemia[86] | Galactose-1-phosphate uridyl transferase*[67], †[34] |
| Gaucher's disease[87] | Glucocerebrosidase[87] |
| Glucose-6-phosphate dehydrogenase deficiency[88] | Glucose-6-phosphate dehydrogenase*[67] |
| Glycogen storage disease type II (Pompe's disease)[89] | $\alpha_1$-4 glucosidase*[67, 70] |
| Homocystinuria[72] | Cystathionine synthase*[72] |
| Marfan's syndrome[90] | Metachromatic granules |
| Mucopolysaccharidosis[77] | Metachromatic granules†[34] |
| Orotic aciduria[91] | Orotidylic pyrophosphorylase and orotidylic decarboxylase |
| Phytanic acid storage disease (Refsum's disease)[92] | Phytanic acid α-hydroxylase*[93] |
| Sphingomyelinosis (Niemann-pick varients)[94] | Sphingomyelinase and/or sphingomyelin and cholesteral accumulation |
| X-linked uric aciduria (Lesch-Nyhan syndrome)[96] | Hypoxanthine quanine phosphoribosyl transferase*[68, 73], †[76] |

*Enzyme present in cultivated amniotic fluid cell.
†Disorder detected in cultivated amniotic fluid cell.

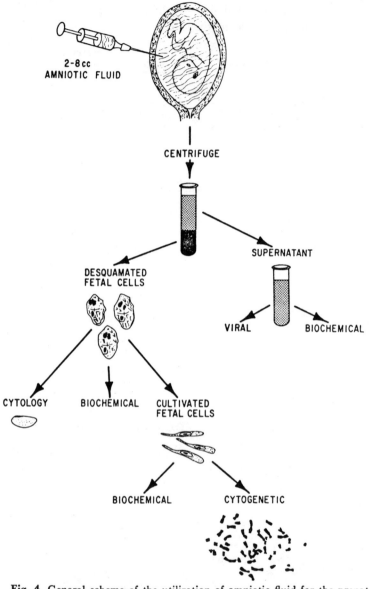

**Fig. 4.** General scheme of the utilization of amniotic fluid for the prenatal detection of genetic disorders.

strate differences of acid phosphatase, alkaline phosphatase, and 6-phosphogluconic dehydrogenase.[67] When glucose-6-phosphate dehydrogenase was studied, a more rapidly migrating extra band was demonstrated in

162

cells derived from two female fetuses at 10 weeks of gestation. One possible explanation for this extra band is that it represents an embryonic form of glucose-6-phosphate dehydrogenase. Qualitative changes of lactate dehydrogenase in cultivated amniotic fluid cells, consisting of a relative increase of $LDH_5$ associated with increased migration toward the cathode, have been found to vary directly with the duration of fetal gestation.[67] Wiggert and Villee[75] have shown that multiple molecular forms of lactic dehydrogenase are present during fetal development and are affected by tissue distribution and age of the fetus.

The prenatal detection of a number of familial metabolic disorders utilizing cultivated amniotic fluid cells has been reported.[34, 76] The in utero diagnosis of a mucopolysaccharidosis was established utilizing the technique of Danes and Bearn[77] to demonstrate the presence of metachromatic granules in cultivated amniotic fluid cells obtained at 28 weeks of fetal gestation.[34] The diagnosis was confirmed after delivery by the demonstration of metachromatic granules in cultured fibroblasts derived from a skin biopsy obtained at seven days of age and the finding of increased urinary excretion of acid mucopolysaccharides. Cultivated amniotic fluid cells obtained immediately prior to cesarean section at 33 weeks of pregnancy in a known heterozygote for galactosemia failed to demonstrate detectable levels of galactose-1-phosphate uridyl transferase. This finding corroborated the lack of galactose-1-phosphate uridyl transferase in cord blood and confirmed the diagnosis of galactosemia.[34] In another case, amniotic fluid cells, obtained at 16 weeks of pregnancy from a known carrier of glycogen storage disease type II (Pompe's disease), demonstrated normal levels of $\alpha$-glucosidase.[34] A healthy male infant was delivered at term having normal levels of leucocyte α-glucosidase. Amniotic fluid cells obtained from a known carrier of maple syrup urine disease at 17 weeks of fetal gestation contained normal levels of α-keto-isocaproate decarboxylase.[71] A healthy female infant was delivered at term; at the age of 2½ months, she had developed normally and had had no detectable amino-aciduria. Uhlendorf and Fujimoto[76] cultivated amniotic fluid cells obtained from a known heterozygote for X-linked uric aciduria (Lesch-Nyhan syndrome). They were able to demonstrate the presence of equal numbers of enzyme deficient and normal cells, establishing that the fetus was a female heterozygous for this X-linked recessive disorder.

The familial metabolic disorders which have been or are potentially capable of intrauterine detection using cultivated amniotic fluid cells are listed in Table II.

Future work must carefully define the "normal characteristics" of cultivated amniotic fluid cells. The presence or absence of embryonic or fetal enzymes, as well as the quantitative and the qualitative changes of enzymes at different stages of fetal gestation, must be determined if this material is to be correctly interpreted.

**Selection and management of high risk pregnancies.** The intrauterine detection of genetic disorders brings a new precision to genetic counseling. The physician may inform the parents that they will have either an affected or a normal child. The risks are no longer one in four, but are 100 per cent or 0. The knowledge that a mother is carrying a fetus with a 100 per cent chance of having a severe defect raises the question of the termination of pregnancy. Although numerous moral, ethical, and legal questions are raised when therapeutic abortion is considered, these problems will not be discussed in this review.

164

Intrauterine treatment of genetic disorders has been limited to the management of Rh iso-immunization. The ability to determine the status of the fetus in utero should stimulate the development of new approaches and techniques of treatment to prevent the intrauterine sequelae of the disease.

The selection of patients for prenatal detection of genetic disorders is currently limited predominantly by the relatively few laboratories working in this area. At the present time, the procedure could be made available to known carriers of either chromosomal aberrations or the inborn errors of metabolism listed in Table II. One might also consider the use of the procedure in women who become pregnant after the age of 40 years. The risk of the procedure in this last group is probably less than the risk of a chromosomal aberration in the fetus.

### SUMMARY

The background and present knowledge of the prenatal detection of genetic defects are reviewed. The general scheme for the utilization of amniotic fluid in prenatal detection of genetic defects is summarized in Fig. 4. A number of cytogenetic and biochemical disorders are capable of detection in utero at the present time. *However, until considerably more experience is gained with these techniques, these procedures should be considered experimental in nature.* Further investigations are needed to define the normal parameters of amniotic fluid and cultivated amniotic fluid cells in order to maximally utilize this material for the prenatal detection of genetic disorders.

I thank Anita Messina, Janet Pi, Greta Shriner, Marilyn Swae, and Janice Wodnicki for tchnical assistance, Dr. David Y.-Y. Hsia and Dr. Robert B. Lawson for their encourage-

ment and critical evaluation, and Lillemor Clever
for help in preparing this manuscript.

## REFERENCES

1. Garrod, A. E.: Inborn errors of metabolism
   (Croonian Lectures), Lancet 2: 1, 73, 142,
   214, 1908.
2. Perry, T. L., Hansen, S., and MacDougall,
   L.: Urinary screening tests in the prevention
   of mental deficiency, Canad. M. A. J. 95:
   89, 1966.
3. Scriver, C. R.: Screening newborns for hereditary metabolic disease, Pediat. Clin. North
   America 12: 807, 1965.
4. Holzel, A. K., Komrower, G. M., and
   Schwarz, V.: Galactosemia, Am. J. Med. 22:
   703, 1957.
5. Synderman, S. E.: Maple syrup urine disease,
   in Nyhan, W. L., editor: Amino acid metabolism and genetic variation, New York, 1967,
   McGraw-Hill Book Company, p. 171.
6. Wilkins, L.: The diagnosis of the adrenogenital syndrome and its treatment with cortisone,
   J. PEDIAT. 41: 860, 1952.
7. Jervis, G. A.: Phenylketonuria, in Nyhan, W.
   L., editor: Amino acid metabolism and genetic variation, New York, 1967, McGraw-
   Hill Book Company, p. 5.
8. Stanbury, J. B., Wyngaarden, J. B., and Fredrickson, D. S.: The metabolic basis of inherited disease, ed 2, New York, 1966, Mc-
   Graw-Hill Book Company.
9. Hsia, D. Y. Y.: Inborn errors of metabolism,
   ed. 2, Chicago, 1966, Year Book Medical
   Publishers, Inc.
10. Harris, H.: Human biochemical genetics,
    London, England, 1959, Cambridge Univer-
    sity Press.
11. Tjio, J. H., and Levan, A.: The chromosome
    number in man, Hereditas 42: 1, 1956.
12. Lejeune, J., Gautier, M., and Turpin, R.:
    Etude des chromosomes somatique de neuf
    enfants mongoliens, Compt. rend. Acad. Sc.
    248: 1821, 1959.
13. Penrose, L. S., Ellis, J. R., and Delhanty, J.
    D. S.: Familial Langdon-Down anomaly with
    chromosomal fusion, Ann. Human Genet. 25:
    243, 1961.
14. Carter, C. O., Hmerton, J. L., Polani, P. E.,
    Gunalp, A., and Weller, S. D. W.: Chromo-
    some translocation as a cause of familial
    mongolism, Lancet 2: 678, 1960.
15. Liley, A. W.: The use of amniocentesis and
    fetal transfusion in erythroblastosis fetalis,
    Pediatrics 35: 836, 1965.
16. Freda, V. J.: Recent obstetrical advances in

the Rh problem. Antepartum management, amniocentesis, and experience with hysterotomy, and surgery in utero, Bull. New York Acad. Med. 42: 474, 1966.

17. Lucey, J. F.: Diagnosis and treatment: Current indication and results of fetal transfusions, Pediatrics 41: 139, 1968.

18. Menees, T. O., Miller, J. D., and Holley, L. E.: Amniography; preliminary report, Am. J. Roentgenol. 24: 363, 1930.

19. Brevis, D. C. A.: Composition of liquor amnii in haemolytic disease of newborn, J. Obst. & Gynaec. Brit. Commonwealth 60: 244, 1953.

20. Liley, A. W.: Liquor amnii analysis in management of pregnancy complicated by rhesus sensitization, Am. J. Obst. & Gynec. 82: 1359, 1961.

21. Freda, V. J.: Rh problem in obstetrics and the new concept of its management using amniocentesis and spectrophotometric scanning of amniotic fluid, Am. J. Obst. & Gynec. 92: 341, 1965.

22. Queenan, J. T.: Amniocentesis and transamniotic fetal transfusion for Rh disease, Clin. Obst. & Gynec. 9: 440, 1966.

23. Burnett, R. G., and Anderson, W. R.: The hazards of amniocentesis, J. Iowa M. Soc. 5f: 130, 1958.

24. Liley, A. W.: Technique and complications of amniocentesis, New Zealand M. J. 59: 581, 1960.

25. Creasman, W. T., Lawrence, R. A., and Thiede, H. A.: Fetal complications of amniocentesis, J. A. M. A. 204: 91, 1968.

26. Berner, H. W., Jr.: Amniography: An accurate way to localize the placenta, Obst. & Gynec. 29: 200, 1967.

27. Wiltchik, S. G., Schwartz, R. H., and Emich, J. D.: Amniography for placental localization, Obst. & Gynec. 28: 641, 1966.

28. Queenan, J. T., and Adams, D. W.: Amniocentesis. A possible immunizing hazard, Obst. & Gynec. 24: 530, 1964.

29. Walker, A. H. C., and Jennison, R. F.: Antenatal prediction of hemolytic disease of newborn. Comparison of liquor amnii and serological studies, Brit. M. J. 2: 1152, 1962.

30. Fairweather, D. V. I., Murray, S., Parkin, D., and Walker, W.: Possible immunological implication of amniocentesis, Lancet 2: 1190, 1963.

31. Cassady, G., Cailleteau, J., Lockard, D., and Milstead, R.: The hazard of fetal-maternal transfusion after transabdominal amniocentesis, Am. J. Obst. & Gynec. 99: 284, 1967.

32. Jacobson, C. B., and Barter, R. H.: Intrauterine diagnosis and management of genetic defects, Am. J. Obst. & Gynec. 99: 796, 1967.

167

33. Fuchs, F.: Genetic information from amniotic fluid constituents, Clin. Obst. & Gynec. 9: 565, 1966.
34. Nadler, H. L.: Antenatal detection of hereditary disorders, Pediatrics. In press.
35. Jacobson, C. B.: Prenatal detection of genetic disease, Joseph P. Kennedy Jr. Foundation, Fourth International Science Symposium on Mental Retardation, Chicago, 1968. In press.
36. Jacobson, C. B. Personal communication.
37. Wagner, G., and Fuchs, F.: The volume of amniotic fluid in the first half of human pregnancy, J. Obst. & Gynaec. Brit. Commonwealth 69: 131, 1962.
38. Plentl, A. A.: Formation and circulation of amniotic fluid, Clin. Obst. & Gynec. 9: 427, 1966.
39. Jacoby, H. E.: Amniotic fluid volumes, Develop. Med. & Child. Neurol. 8: 587, 1966.
40. Bonsnes, R. W.: Composition of amniotic fluid, Clin. Obst. & Gynec. 9: 440, 1966.
41. Seppälä, M., Ruoslahti, E., and Tallberg, T. H.: Genetical evidence for maternal origin of amniotic fluid proteins, Ann. med. exper. et biol. Fenniae 44: 6, 1966.
42. Dancis, J., Lind, J., and Vera, P.: In Villee, C. A. editor: The placenta and foetal membranes, Baltimore, 1960, The Williams & Wilkins Company, p. 185.
43. Brzezinski, A., Sadovsky, E., and Shafrir, E.: Electrophoretic distribution of proteins in amniotic fluid and in maternal and fetal serum, Am. J. Obst. & Gynec. 82: 800, 1961.
44. Brzezinski, A., Sadovsky, E., and Shafrir, E.: Protein composition of early amniotic fluid and fetal serum with a case of bis-albuminemia, Am. J. Obst. & Gynec. 89: 488, 1964.
45. Jeffcoate, T. N. A., Fliegner, J. R. H., Russell, S. H., Davis, J. C., and Wade, A P.: Diagnosis of adrenogenital syndrome before birth, Lancet 2: 553, 1965.
46. Fuchs, F.: Discussion of paper by Jacobson and Barter, Am. J. Obst. & Gynec. 99: 806, 1967.
47. Graven, S. N.: Phospholipids in human and monkey amniotic fluid, The Society for Pediatric Research Program and Abstracts, Atlantic City, New Jersey, 1968, p. 52.
48. Graven, S. N., Opitz, J. M., and Harrison, M.: The respiratory distress syndrome, Am. J. Obst. & Gynec. 96: 969, 1966.
49. Van Leeuwen, L., Jacoby, H., and Charles, D.: Exfoliative cytology of amniotic fluid, Acta cytol. 9: 442, 1965.
50. Fuchs, F., and Riis, P.: Antenatal sex determination, Nature 177: 330, 1956.
51. Shettles, L. B.: Nuclear morphology of cells

168

in amniotic fluid in relation to sex of infant, Am. J. Obst. & Gynec. **71:** 834, 1956.

52. Makowski, E. L., Prem, K. A., and Kaiser, I. H.: Detection of sex of fetuses by the incidence of sex chromatin body in nuclei of cells in amniotic fluid, Science **123:** 542, 1956.

53. Serr, D. M., Sachs, L., and Danon, M.: Diagnosis of sex before birth using cells from amniotic fluid, Bull. Res. Council Israel 5B137, 1955.

54. Dewhurst, C. J.: Diagnosis of sex before birth, Lancet **1:** 471, 1956.

55. James, F.: Sexing foetuses by examination of the amniotic fluid, Lancet **1:** 202, 1956.

56. Keymer, E., Silva-Inzunza, E., and Coutts, W. E.: Contribution to the antenatal determination of sex, Am. J. Obst. & Gynec. **74:** 1098, 1957.

57. Pasquinucci, C.: Studio della "Chromatina sessuale" nelle cellule del liquido amniotico per la diagnosi prenatale di sesso, Ann. Obst. & Ginec. **79:** 152, 1957.

58. Amarose, A. P., Wallingford, A. J., and Plotz, E. J.: Prediction of fetal sex from cytologic examination of amniotic fluid, New England J. Med. **275:** 715, 1966.

59. Riis, P., and Fuchs, F.: Sex chromatin and antenatal sex diagnosis, *in* Moore, K. G., editor: The sex chromatin, Philadelphia, 1966, W. B. Saunders Company.

60. Serr, D. M., and Margolis, E.: Diagnosis of fetal sex in a sex-linked hereditary disorder, Am. J. Obst. & Gynec. **88:** 230, 1964.

61. Fuchs, F., Freiesleben, E., Knudsen, E. E., and Riis, P.: Determination of foetal bloodgroup, Lancet **1:** 996, 1956.

62. Sachs, L., Feldman, M., and Danon, M.: Prenatal identification of blood group antigens, Lancet **2:** 356, 1956.

63. Broussy, J., Ducos, J., and Baux, R.: Mise en evidence des antigenes A et B dans le liquide amniotique humain et en, Compt. rend. Soc. biol. **152:** 172, 1958.

64. Gordon, H., and Brosens, I.: Cytology of amniotic fluid: A new test for fetal maturity, Obst. & Gynec. **30:** 652, 1967.

65. Steele, M. W., and Breg, W. R.: Chromosome analysis of human amniotic-fluid cells, Lancet **1:** 383, 1966.

66. Thiede, H. A., Creasman, W. T., and Metcalfe, S.: Antenatal analysis of the human chromosomes, Am. J. Obst. & Gynec. **94:** 589, 1966.

67. Nadler, H. L.: Patterns of enzyme development using cultivated human fetal cells from amniotic fluid, Biochem. Genet. **2:** 119, 1968.

169

68. Uhlendorf, B. W., Jacobson, C. B., Sloan, H. R., Mudd, S. H., Herndon, J. H., Brady, R O., Seegmiller, J. E., and Fujimoto, W.: Cell cultures derived from human amniotic fluid: Their possible application in the intra-uterine diagnosis of heritable metabolic disease, Nineteenth Annual Meeting of the Tissue Culture Association, Schedule and Abstracts, San Juan, Puerto Rico, 1968, In Vitro. In press.

69. Dancis, J.: The antepartum diagnosis of genetic diseases, J. PEDIAT. 72: 301, 1968.

70. Dancis, J. Personal communication.

71. Nadler, H. L., and Dancis, J.: Unpublished data.

72. Uhlendorf, B. W., and Mudd, S. H.: Cystathionine synthase in tissue culture derived from human skin: Enzyme defect in homocystinuria, Science 160, 1007, 1968.

73. Berman, P., and Dancis, J.: Personal communication.

74. Nadler, H. L., Dowben, R. M., and Hsia, D. Y.-Y.: Ultra-centrifugal separation of fractions obtained from cells ruptured by nitrogen cavitation. The Society for Pediatric Research, Program and Abstracts, Atlantic City, New Jersey, 1968, p. 101.

75. Wiggert, B. O., and Villee, C. A.: Multiple molecular forms of malic and lactic dehydrogenase during development, J. Biol. Chem. 239: 444, 1964.

76. Uhlendorf, B. W., and Fugimoto, W.: Personal communication.

77. Danes, B. S., and Bearn, A. G.: Hurler's syndrome. A genetic study in cell culture, J. Exper. Med. 123: 1, 1966.

78. Krooth, R. S., Howell, R. R., and Hamilton, H. B.: Properties of acatalasic cells growing in vitro, J. Exper. Med. 115: 313, 1962.

79. Dancis, J., Jansen, V., Hutzler, J., and Levitz, M.: The metabolism of leucine in tissue culture of skin fibroblasts of maple-syrup-urine disease, Biochim. et biophys. acta 77: 523, 1963.

80. Uhlendorf, B. W., and Seegmiller, J. E.: Personal communication.

81. Danes, B. S., and Bearn, A. G.: Cell culture and the Chediak-Higashi syndrome, Lancet 2: 65, 1967.

82. Tedesco, T. A., and Mellman, W. J.: Arginosuccinate synthetase activity and citrulline metabolism in cells cultured from a citrullinemic subject, Proc. Nat. Acad. Sc. 57: 829, 1967.

83. Uhlendorf, B. W., and Mudd, S. H.: Personal communication.

84. Danes, B. S., and Bearn, A. G.: A genetic cell marker in cystic fibrosis of the pancreas,

Lancet 1: 1061, 1968.

85. Schneider, J. A., Rosenbloom, F. M., Bradley, K. H., and Seegmiller, J. E.: Increased free-cystine content of fibroblasts cultured from patients with cystinosis, Biochem. & Biophys. Res. Comm. 29: 527, 1967.

86. Krooth, R. S., and Weinberg, A. N.: Studies on cell lines developed from the tissues of patients with galactosemia, J. Exper. Med. 113: 1155, 1961.

87. Uhlendorf, B. W., and Brady, R. Personal Communication.

88. Davidson, R. G., Nitowsky, H. M., and Childs, B.: Demonstration of two populations of cells in the human female heterozygous for glucose-6-phosphate dehydrogenase variants, Proc. Nat. Acad. Sc. 50: 481, 1963.

89. Nitowsky, H. M., and Grunfeld, A.: Lysosomal α-glucosidase in type II glycogenesis; activity in leucocytes and cell cultures in relation to genotype, J. Lab. & Clin. Med. 69: 472, 1967.

90. Matelon, R., and Dorfman, A.: Mucopolysaccharide abnormality in fibroblasts of the Marfan syndrome, The American Pediatrics Society, Inc., Program and Abstracts, Atlantic City. N. J., 1968, p. 7.

91. Pinsky, L.: and Krooth, R. S.: Studies on the control of pyrimidine biosynthesis in human diploid cell strains. I. Effect of 6-azauridine on cellular phenotype, Proc. Nat. Acad. Sc. 57: 925, 1967.

92. Steinberg, D., Herndon, J. H., Uhlendorf, B. W., Mize, C. E., Avigan, J., and Milne, G. W. A.: Refsum's disease: Nature of the enzyme defect, Science 156: 1740, 1967.

93. Uhlendorf, B. W., and Herndon, J., Jr.: Personal communication.

94. Uhlendorf, B. W., Holtz, A. I., Mock, M. B., and Fredrickson, D. S.: Persistance of a metabolic defect in tissue culture derived from patients with Nieman-Pick disease, in Aronson, S. M., and Volk, B. W., editors: Inborn disorders of sphingolipid metabolism, Oxford, 1967, Pergamon Press, p. 443.

95. Uhlendorf, B. W., and Sloan, H.: Personal Communication.

96. Seegmiller, J. E., Rosenbloom, F. M., and Kelley, W. N.. Enzyme defect associated with a sex-linked human neurological disorder and excessive purine synthesis, Science 155: 1682, 1967.

171

# PRENATAL GENETIC DIAGNOSIS

Aubrey Milunsky, MB.B.Ch., M.R.C.P., John W. Littlefield, M.D.,
Julian N. Kanfer, Ph.D.,   Edwin H. Kolodny, M.D.,

Vivian E. Shih, M.D., and Leonard Atkins, M.D.

THE fear of bearing a deformed or mentally defective child is a universal emotion shared by most women at some time during pregnancy. Usually, sympathetic counsel by the obstetrician suffices to keep the woman's worst fears from surfacing. In the particular cases in which a previous pregnancy resulted in a chromosomally abnormal offspring or one with known genetic disease, simple reassurance may fail, and chronic anxiety or severe depression may supervene. Genetic counseling based upon a method that could accurately diagnose disorders in utero would serve not only to allay many fears but also to prevent, if the parents desire it, the births of many children with mental defect or fatal disease of genetic origin.

The observations by Barr and Bertram,[1] in 1949, of morphologic sex differences in the nerve-cell

Supported by research grants (AM-13655, NB-08994-02 and NB-05096) from the U.S. Public Health Service, and a project (No. 906) from the Maternal and Child Health Service (Dr. Kolodny is the recipient of a special fellowship [2F11 NB1849-02 NSRB] from the National Institute of Neurological Diseases and Stroke).

nuclei of cats set the stage for human sex determination. Fuchs,[2] in 1955, and others[3-6] first showed the feasibility of fetal sex determination from amniotic-fluid cells. A few years later, after successful amniotic-fluid cell culture, it became possible to demonstrate the fetal karyotype by this method.[7,8] Thus far, at least 15 cases of mongolism have been diagnosed prenatally,[8-11] as well as five other fetuses with chromosomal anomalies, including XYY and XXY karyotypes.[11]

Rapid advances in the past decade in somatic cell genetics have made it possible to diagnose an increasing number of disorders by tissue-culture methods.[12] The cultured fibroblast derived from skin has been the most useful cell. The initial steps have been the characterization of certain diseases in cultured skin fibroblasts, which has in general been followed by efforts at making specific prenatal diagnoses with the use of amniotic-fluid cells.

### AMNIOTIC FLUID

The data on the formation and circulation, volume and composition of amniotic fluid have recently been reviewed.[13-16] Although the exact origin and fate of amniotic fluid remains unknown, it is clear that the term fetus swallows about 450 ml of fluid and passes about 500 ml of urine every 24 hours. According to Fuchs, at 14 weeks' gestation the amniotic-fluid volume is between 98 and 116 ml, and at 16 weeks between 208 and 285 ml.[14] At 20 weeks Plentl reports an average amniotic-fluid volume of 350 ml.[13]

The cellular pleomorphism of amniotic fluid seen immediately after amniocentesis resolves in culture over one to four weeks into a cell line which may be predominantly fibroblastic, epithelioid or mixed. The amniotic-fluid cells are of fetal origin, and derived mainly from fetal skin and amnion.[8,17] Successful cultivation of these cells is related to gestational age, being much more likely earlier in pregnancy.[7,18,19] The working hypothesis has emerged that some disorders evident in cultured skin fibroblasts could also be diagnosed in cultured amniotic-fluid cells.

The composition of amniotic fluid resembles that of extracellular fluid. As pregnancy progresses the factors that alter this resemblance to extracellular fluid include deglutition, micturition and defecation.

174

Amino acids are present in amniotic fluid in about the same concentration as in maternal plasma.[15] Fetal urinary excretion of enzymes, amino acids and abnormal metabolites into amniotic fluid provides a ready source of diagnostic material. The origin of proteins in the amniotic fluid has been reported to be maternal by some,[20,21] whereas others have presented evidence of fetal origin.[22,23]

## AMNIOCENTESIS

Transabdominal amniocentesis, long known in relation to induced abortion, became more recently an important tool in the management of Rh disease, and has only lately been used to obtain amniotic fluid for prenatal genetic studies. The technic has gained widespread acceptance in Rh disease,[24,25] since there has been minimal maternal and fetal morbidity or mortality.[26,27]

Over 300 amniocenteses have been done specifically for prenatal genetic studies in high-risk pregnancies.[8,28,29] In the largest series, amniocenteses were successfully performed in 160 of 162 cases, repeat procedures being required in seven.[28] Successful cultivation of amniotic-fluid cells was accomplished in all 155 pregnancies studied. The results of chromosomal analyses on the cultured cells were obtained within an average period of 14 days (range of 15 to 40 days) after amniocentesis.

The value of placental localization before amniocentesis by means of a [51]Cr-tagged red-cell technic has already been shown.[30] The use of ultrasonic placentography[31,32] for placental localization, however, has not been evaluated in patients undergoing amniocentesis early in gestation for prenatal studies. The placenta can be readily identified by ultrasonic detection from the 14th week of gestation.[31] Since the ultrasonic procedure is considered to be safe[33-35] careful assessment should determine its place in amniocentesis in early gestation. In addition, this technic should be useful in determining the presence of twins in patients undergoing amniocentesis.

Transabdominal amniocentesis performed for Rh disease is usually done well after 20 weeks of gestation, and the risk to mother or baby is small.[26,27,36-38] Among reported complications, fetal morbidity appears to be greater than maternal after 20 weeks' gestation. Fetal deaths may result from abruptio

175

placentae, amnionitis and fetal hemorrhage,[27,36,38] and puncture of the fetus has been observed in some cases.[27,39,40] Maternal morbidity has included maternal hemorrhage, abdominal pain and peritonitis.[38] Transvaginal amniocentesis in early pregnancy carries a significant risk of precipitating abortion or infecting the mother and is not advised.[41] Moreover, the likelihood of obtaining a contaminated amniotic-fluid sample further precludes the use of this approach for prenatal diagnostic studies.

Nadler and Gerbie[28] had no maternal or fetal complications in their series of 155 pregnancies, amniocenteses having been done at 13 to 18 weeks' gestation for diagnostic reasons. They also have information that a further 132 patients have had amniocenteses for prenatal genetic studies in three other centers, all without fetal or maternal morbidity or mortality. It is, nevertheless, too early to make an accurate assessment of the degree of inherent risk of amniocentesis done between 13 and 18 weeks of gestation. It seems that the procedure is too hazardous earlier than 14 weeks' gestation, in view of the small amount of amniotic fluid available in relation to fetal and uterine size. Our own present policy is to perform the procedure selectively at 16 weeks' gestation as recommended by Nadler.[19] Others, however, have advocated the procedure as early as 14 weeks' gestation.[42] Perhaps the ideal timing of amniocentesis could best be based on the presence of a certain minimum amniotic-fluid volume rather than gestational age, if such a method to determine this volume could be devised simply and safely.

The strict adherence to aseptic technic during the amniocentesis should be extended to include transfer of the fluid into a specially prepared sterile siliconized container. Although it is best to culture the fetal cells as soon after the procedure as possible, the sample can be refrigerated overnight or sent airmail. The greatest care should be exercised to obtain safe transportation and delivery of these samples obtained at risk to mother and fetus.

In the overall evaluation of this technic, the possibility of late sequelae will require attention. In the report of 160 amniocenteses in 155 pregnancies by Nadler and Gerbie,[28] seven infants weighed less than 2100 g (4 lb, 10 oz) at birth. It was not stated whether these infants were truly premature or small for dates. Further studies could establish the frequency (if any) of initiating or aggravating maternal sensitization to fetal blood admixture, and the risk (if any) of congenital or "acquired" fetal deformity.

Biopsy of the placenta in early pregnancy has already been achieved,[43] and skin biopsy of the fetus in utero was recently performed in eight women in the second or third trimester of pregnancy[44] within 10 days before therapeutic abortion. The procedure was done "blind," and faintly visible stab wounds were found on the cheek and forehead in two of four fetuses. In our view the especially hazardous nature of the "blind" technic described precludes its further use without modification.

A tentative classification of pregnancies appropriate for amniocentesis was recently proposed by one of us (J.W.L.) in the *Journal,* on the basis of the severity of the disorder and the degree of genetic risk,[45] and the decision was always predicated on the ultimate desire of the family for this test as well as for any subsequent intervention.[46] In this paper, we have considered the disorders that, with our present knowledge, can possibly and usefully be diagnosed before birth under the broad categories of chromosomal aberrations, sex-linked diseases, metabolic disorders and a miscellaneous group of diseases (Table 1).

## CHROMOSOMAL ABERRATIONS

Significant chromosomal abnormalities have been estimated to occur once in every 200 live births,[143] and include Down's, Turner's, and Klinefelter's syndromes, trisomy 18, trisomy 13-15, cri-du-chat syndrome, triple-X females, XYY males, D/G and other translocations, certain other deletions and autosomal and sex chromosome syndromes. It is known that the prevalence of the commoner autosomal trisomies (trisomy 21, trisomy 13-15, and trisomy 18) and sex chromosome aneuploidies (47 XXY, 47 XXX and 47 XYY) rises with increasing maternal age.[144-146] The incidence of trisomy 21 (mongolism), for example, is about 1:2300 under the age of 20 years, 1:290 from 35 to 39 years, and 1:100 from 40 to 44 years and rises to about 1:46 at 45 years of age and over.[147,148] The numerical importance alone is apparent when the prevalence of children with trisomy 21 born to mothers over the age of 35 is considered. In general, these older

Table 1. Prenatal Diagnosis of Hereditary Metabolic Disorders by Amniocentesis.

| DISORDERS* | MAJOR CLINICAL MANIFESTATIONS | ACCUMULATED PRODUCTS OR OTHER FEATURES IN TISSUES OR CULTURED FIBROBLASTS | DEFICIENT ENZYME ACTIVITY OR OTHER FEATURE IN TISSUES OR CULTURED FIBROBLASTS |
|---|---|---|---|
| Disorders of lipid metabolism: | | | |
| Fabry's disease*[47-50] | Purple skin papules; renal failure; cardiac & ocular involvement. | Ceramidetrihexoside | Ceramidetrihexoside galactosidase |
| Gaucher's disease[51,52] | Infantile & adult forms; hepatosplenomegaly, erosion of long bones, neurologic involvement, anemia & thrombocytopenia. | Glucocerebroside | Glucocerebrosidase |
| G$_{M1}$ gangliosicosis (generalized gangliosidosis)[53-58] | Mental retardation from birth; unusual facies; hepatosplenomegaly & skeletal changes. | G$_{M1}$ ganglioside & ceramide tetrahexoside; visceral mucopolysaccharide of keratan sulfate type & a sialomucopolysaccharide. | Beta-galactosidase A, B & C; B & C only. |
| G$_{M2}$ gangliosidosis (Tay–Sachs disease)[53,59-65] | Onset at age of 5 to 6 mo; degenerative neurologic disorder with cherry-red spot within macula progressing from normal to apathy, hypotonia, profound psychomotor retardation & death. | G$_{M2}$ ganglioside & its asialo derivative | Hexosaminidase A

Hexosaminidase A & B |
| Metachromatic leukodystrophy[66-70] | At least 2 forms: degenerative neurologic disease progressing from normal to weakness, ataxia, hypotonia, mental retardation & paralysis; & excessive sulfatide in urine. | Sulfatide | Arylsulfatase A (sulfatidase) |
| Niemann–Pick disease[2,71-74] | 4 types: hepatosplenomegaly & variable skeletal & neurologic involvement | Sphingomyelin | Sphingomyelinase |
| Refsum's disease[75-77] | Cerebellar ataxia; peripheral polyneuropathy; retinitis pigmentosa; & other cardiac, skin, neurologic & skeletal changes. | Phytanic acid | Phytanic acid alpha-hydroxylase |
| Mucopolysaccharidoses: | | | |
| Hurler's syndrome[78-84] | Gargoyle-like facies; early clouding of cornea; early | Dermatan sulfate & heparitin sulfate | Specific beta-galactosidase |

178

| Disorder | Clinical features | | |
|---|---|---|---|
| Hunter's syndrome*[80,82,83,85] | psychomotor retardation; increased linear growth in 1st yr; then decline to become dwarfed; hepatosplenomegaly; kyphosis; joint stiffness; excessive dermatan sulfate & heparitin sulfate in urine. | As in Hurler's syndrome | Unknown |
| | Gargoyle-like facies less obvious & seen later than in Hurler's syndrome; clear cornea; psychomotor retardation; increased linear growth in 1st yr, will decline later; hepatosplenomegaly; joint stiffness; excessive dermatan sulfate & heparitin sulfate in urine. | | |
| Maroteaux–Lamy syndrome[80] | Severe skeletal changes; cloudy corneas; normal intellect; excessive dermatan sulfate in urine. | Unknown | Unknown |
| Morquio's syndrome[80] | Severe skeletal changes, with dwarfism; cloudy corneas; aortic regurgitation; intellect usually within normal range; excessive keratan sulfate in urine. | Unknown | Unknown |
| Sanfilippo syndrome[80,82] | Severe mental retardation; joint stiffness; excessive heparitin sulfate in urine. | Unknown | Unknown |
| Scheie's syndrome[80] | Coarse facies; stiff joints; usually normal intellect; aortic regurgitation; excessive dermatan sulfate in urine. | Unknown | Unknown |
| Amino acid & related disorders: | | | |
| Argininosuccinic aciduria[86,87] | Mental retardation; trichorrhexis nodosa; ammonia intoxication. | Argininosuccinic acid | Argininosuccinase |

*All disorders listed are autosomal recessive, except for those marked * (X-linked recessive) or † (autosomal dominant).

Table 1 (Continued).

| Location of Enzyme or Other Feature | Location of Enzyme Deficiency or Other Abnormality | Prenatal Diagnosis |
|---|---|---|
| Cultured skin fibroblast | Cultured skin fibroblast | Potentially possible in future |
| Cultured skin fibroblast; cultured amniotic-fluid cell. | Cultured skin fibroblast | Possible |
| Cultured skin fibroblast; cultured amniotic fluid cell; amniotic fluid. | Cultured skin fibroblast | Possible |
| Cultured skin fibroblast; cultured amniotic-fluid cell; noncultured amniotic-fluid cell; amniotic fluid. | Cultured skin fibroblast; noncultured amniotic-fluid cell. | Made |
| Cultured skin fibroblast; cultured amniotic-fluid cell. | Cultured skin fibroblast | Possible |
| Cultured skin fibroblast; cultured amniotic-fluid cell. | Cultured skin fibroblast; cultured amniotic-fluid cell. | Made |
| Cultured skin fibroblast; cultured amniotic-fluid cell. | Cultured skin fibroblast; cultured amniotic-fluid cell. | Made |
| Cultured skin fibroblast; cultured amniotic-fluid cell. | Cultured skin fibroblast | Possible |
| Cultured skin fibroblast; cultured amniotic-fluid cell; | Cultured skin fibroblast; cultured amniotic-fluid cell; | Made |

| | | |
|---|---|---|
| amniotic fluid. | amniotic fluid. | |
| Unknown | Cultured skin fibroblast; cultured amniotic-fluid cell; amniotic fluid. | Potentially possible in future |
| Cultured skin fibroblast | Unknown | Potentially possible in future |
| Cultured skin fibroblast | Unknown | Potentially possible in future |
| Unknown | Unknown | Potentially possible in future |
| Cultured skin fibroblast; cultured amniotic-fluid cell. | Cultured skin fibroblast | Possible |

181

Table 1 (Continued).

| DISORDERS* | MAJOR CLINICAL MANIFESTATIONS | ACCUMULATED PRODUCTS OR OTHER FEATURES IN TISSUES OR CULTURED FIBROBLASTS | DEFICIENT ENZYME ACTIVITY OR OTHER FEATURE IN TISSUES OR CULTURED FIBROBLASTS |
|---|---|---|---|
| Citrullinemia[88] | Ammonia intoxication; mental retardation. | Citrulline | Argininosuccinic acid synthetase |
| Cystinosis[89-91] | Failure to thrive; rickets; glycosuria; aminoaciduria; cystine deposition in tissue. | Cystine | Unknown |
| Homocystinuria[92] | Dislocated lenses; skeletal abnormalities; vascular thrombosis; mental retardation. | Methionine & homocystine | Cystathionine synthase |
| Hyperammonemia, Type II[93] | Ammonia intoxication; mental retardation. | Ornithine carbamyl-transferase | Ornithine carbamyl transferase |
| Hyperlysinemia[94] | Mental retardation; muscular asthenia (may be normal). | Lysine | Lysine-ketoglutarate reductase |
| Hypervalinemia[18] | Mental retardation; failure to thrive. | Valine | Valine transaminase |
| Ketotic hyper-glycinemia[95] | Ketoacidosis; protein intolerance; developmental retardation. | Glycine | Proprionyl CoA carboxylase |
| Maple-syrup-urine disease: Severe infantile[11,96-99] | Ketoacidosis; neurologic abnormality; mental retardation; early death. | Valine, leucine, isoleucine, alloiso-leucine | Branched-chain keto acid decarboxylase |
| Intermittent[96,99] | Ketoacidosis; neurologic abnormality; mental retardation; early death. | As above | As above |
| Methylmalonic aciduria[11,100-102] | Acidosis; lethargy; failure to thrive; early death. | Methylmalonic acid, glycine, homocystine, & cystathionine | Methylmalonyl CoA isomerase or vitamin $B_{12}$ coenzyme (decreased carbon dioxide production from propionate) |
| Ornithine-alpha-ketoacid transaminase deficiency[103] | Liver disease; renal tubular defect; mental retardation. | Ornithine | Ornithine-alpha-keto acid transaminase |
| Disorders of carbohydrate metabolism: Fucosidosis[104-106] | Severe progressive cerebral | Fucose containing hetero- | Alpha-fucosidase |

182

| | polysaccharide | degeneration; intense spasticity; thick skin & excessive sweating; increased salinity of sweat. | |
| --- | --- | --- | --- |
| Glycogen-storage disease (Type II)[107-110] | Glycogen storage | Failure to thrive; hypotonia; hepatomegaly; cardiomegaly. | Alpha-1, 4-glucosidase |
| Glycogen-storage disease (Type III)[111] | Abnormally structured glycogen | Hepatomegaly; cardiomegaly; hypoglycemia. | Amylo-1, 6-glucosidase |
| Glycogen-storage disease (Type IV)[111] | Abnormally structured glycogen | Familial cirrhosis with splenomegaly | Branching enzyme |
| Galactosemia[112-114] | Galactose | Cirrhosis, cataracts, mental retardation & failure to thrive. | Galactose-1-P uridyl transferase |
| Mannosidosis[106a,115,116] | Mannose and glucosamine containing heteropolysaccharide | Gargoyle-like facies; psychomotor retardation; accelerated growth in infancy; hypotonia; mild hepatosplenomegaly. | Alpha-mannosidase |
| Pyruvate decarboxylase[117,118] deficiency | Pyruvic acid, alanine and lactate | Intermittent cerebellar ataxia & choreoathetosis, with elevated urinary alanine | Pyruvate decarboxylase deficiency |
| Glucose-6-PO$_4$ dehydrogenase[19] deficiency | – | Hemolytic anemia | G-6-PO$_4$ dehydrogenase |
| Miscellaneous disorders: Acatalasemia[120] | Unknown | Recurrent & anaerobic infections of gums & oral tissue | Catalase |
| Adrenogenital syndrome[12-125] | – | Virilization or pseudohermaphrodism; adrenal insufficiency, with salt loss; hypertensive cardiovascular disease; pregnanetriol & 17-ketosteroids in urine. | Failure of C21, C11 or steroid hydroxylation |

Table 1 (Continued).

| LOCATION OF ENZYME OR OTHER FEATURE | LOCATION OF ENZYME DEFICIENCY OR OTHER ABNORMALITY | PRENATAL DIAGNOSIS |
|---|---|---|
| Cultured skin fibroblast | Cultured skin fibroblast | Potentially possible in future |
| Cultured skin fibroblast; cultured amniotic-fluid cell. | Cultured skin fibroblast | Possible |
| Cultured skin fibroblast; cultured amniotic-fluid cell. | Cultured skin fibroblast | Possible |
| Noncultured amniotic-fluid cell | None present | Possible |
| Cultured skin fibroblast | Cultured skin fibroblast | Potentially possible in future |
| Cultured skin fibroblast | None present | Potentially possible in future |
| Cultured skin fibroblast | Cultured skin fibroblast | Potentially possible in future |
| Cultured skin fibroblast; cultured amniotic-fluid cell. | Cultured skin fibroblast; cultured amniotic-fluid cell. | Made |
| Cultured skin fibroblast; cultured amniotic-fluid cell. | Cultured skin fibroblast; cultured amniotic-fluid cell. | Possible |
| Cultured skin fibroblast; cultured amniotic-fluid cell. | Cultured skin fibroblast; amniotic fluid. | Made |
| Cultured skin fibroblast; cultured amniotic-fluid cell. | None present | Possible |
| Cultured skin fibroblast; cul- | None present | Potentially possible in future |

184

turec amniotic-fluid cell.

| | | |
|---|---|---|
| Cultured skin fibroblast; cultured amniotic-fluid cell; non-cultured amniotic fluid cell amniotic fluid | Cultured skin fibroblast; cultured amniotic-fluid cell; noncultured amniotic-fluid cell; amniotic fluid. | Made |
| | None present | Possible |
| Cultured skin fibroblast; cultured amniotic-fluid cell. | Cultured skin fibroblast | Possible |
| Cultured skin fibroblast; cultured amniotic-fluid cell. | Cultured skin fibroblast; cultured amniotic-fluid cell; noncultured amniotic-fluid cell. | Made |
| Cultured skin fibroblast; cultured amniotic-fluid cell; noncultured amniotic-fluid cell. | None present | Possible |
| Cultured skin fibroblast; cultured amniotic-fluid cell. | | |
| Cultured skin fibroblast | None present | Potentially possible in future |
| Cultured skin fibroblast; cultured amniotic-fluid cell; noncultured amniotic-fluid cell. | Cultured skin fibroblast | Possible |
| Cultured skin fibroblast | None present | Potentially possible in future |
| Amniotic fluid | Amniotic fluid | Made |

Table 1 (Continued).

| Disorders* | Major Clinical Manifestations | Accumulated Products or Other Features in Tissues or Cultured Fibroblasts | Deficient Enzyme Activity or Other Feature in Tissues or Cultured Fibroblasts |
|---|---|---|---|
| Chediak–Higashi syndrome[126] | Photobia; decreased pigmentation of skin, hair & eyes; increased susceptibility to infections. | Cellular inclusions | Unknown |
| Congenital erythropoietic porphyria[50,127] | Photosensitive dermatitis; anemia; splenomegaly; hypertrichosis; & massive porphyrinuria. | Uroporphyrin I and coproporphyrin I in tissues | Cosynthetase |
| Cystic fibrosis[128–132] | Recurrent pulmonary infection; malabsorption; failure to thrive. | Mucopolysaccharide storage or increased production in cultured fibroblasts | Beta-glucuronidase deficiency in skin components |
| I-cell disease[133–136] | Gargoyle-like facies; dwarfism from birth; gingival hyperplasia; psychomotor retardation. | Acid mucopolysaccharide and glycolipids | Reduced beta-glucuronidase & excessive acid phosphatase |
| Lesch–Nyhan syndrome*[136,137] | Self mutilation; choreoathetosis; spasticity; mental retardation. | Uric acid | Hypoxanthine-guanine phosphoribosyltransferase |
| Lysosomal acid phosphatase deficiency[138] | Failure to thrive; progressive neuromuscular involvement; hypoglycemia; seizures & hepatomegaly. | Unknown | Lysosomal acid phosphatase |
| Marfan's syndrome†[139] | Connective-tissue disorder, with skeletal, cardiovascular & ocular signs | Hyaluronic acid in cultured fibroblasts | Unknown |
| Orotic aciduria[11,140] | Infantile megaloblastic anemia; orotic acid in urine. | Unknown | Orotidylic pyrophosphorylase & decarboxylase |
| Xeroderma pigmentosum[141,142] | Photosensitive dermatitis & skin cancers | Unknown | DNA "repair enzyme" |

*All disorders listed are autosomal recessive, except for those marked * (X-linked recessive) or † (autosomal dominant).

mothers constitute only 13.5 per cent of all pregnancies, but they produce over 50 per cent of all infants with mongolism.[149]

Familial mongolism may result from the translocation of part of a number 21 chromosome to another chromosome. The incidence of D/G and G/G translocation is 2 to 3 per cent and 1.2 per cent respectively of all children with mongolism.[149,150] A 21/21 (G/G) translocation carrier has a 100 per cent risk of having an affected child.[151] In contrast, a female D/G heterozygote runs a 9 per cent risk of having another child with mongolism, and for a male heterozygote the risk is about 4 per cent, and may even be lower.[152] For 21/22 translocation carriers the available information suggests a recurrence risk for mongolism of about 5 per cent.[153] For both these translocations the apparent risk for both male and female heterozygotes is very much less than the theoretically expected 33 per cent recurrence risk.[153,154] In D/D translocation carriers the risk of having children with an unbalanced chromosome complement is less than 1 per cent.[153] The frequency of children with unbalanced chromosome complements born to patients with reciprocal translocations appears to be lower than the theoretical 50 per cent.[155,156] In most cases chromosomal analysis after amniocentesis can now distinguish the affected from the carrier or normal fetus in this situation, as well as in other familial chromosome disorders.

The cytogenetic study of cultured and noncultured amniotic-fluid cells has become an established and practical diagnostic method.[7-9,157] Provided that control of high quality is exercised, both fetal sex and karyotype can be accurately determined. Fuchs[2] and others[3-6] have demonstrated the ease and accuracy with which fetal sex can be determined. Our procedure is first to assess the sex-chromatin masses (Barr bodies) in the amniotic-fluid cells that fail to attach to the dish after 24 hours in culture. Preparations of these desquamated cells for sex-chromatin studies may not always be satisfactory. Nelson and Emery[158] found that accurate sex prediction was possible in only 91 per cent of cases, the other cell preparations being of too poor quality for reliable comment. Study of the desquamated cells provides a rapid answer for the fetal sex, but a double check should be made with the karyotype derived later from the cultured cells. Errors in sex or karyotype

187

determination may occur. With twins only one amniotic sac may be aspirated, the presence of the other twin being missed. Maternal cells may inadvertently be obtained with the needle or through maternal-blood admixture. Nadler and Gerbie mentioned two cases in which maternal cells may have been obtained,[28] and suggest that if cultured amniotic-fluid cells grow rapidly almost immediately, presence of maternal cells must be suspected. It is possible that a phenotypically male fetus may be chromatin positive. Accumulated sex-chromatin studies of buccal smears from newborn infants have shown that of 16,089 females, 1:3018 (0.03 per cent) was chromatin negative.[159] This is an additional reason to check the fetal sex by means of the karyotype from cultured amniotic-fluid cells. It is self-evident that in view of the critical nature of the anticipated result, the greatest care and caution be exercised in the interpretation of the karyotype. Nadler[28] notes one case in which an error in reading the karyotypic sex was made.

In 16 consecutive amniocenteses, we have noted tetraploidy occurring regularly in the cultured amniotic-fluid cells, with a frequency varying up to 43 per cent, the remaining metaphase spreads being mostly normal. Observations made on the basis of sex-chromatin studies and cellular DNA determinations[160] indicated that tetraploid cells occur naturally in the human amnion, and these results have had further confirmation.[161] Schlegel et al., in studying structurally normal aborted amnions,[162] found tetraploidy in 10 per cent of the total cells counted, and indicated that they were not concentrated in a few specimens but were randomly distributed throughout the series. It could be argued that tetraploidy may be an artifactual consequence of tissue culture. However, from the studies of Shlegel et al.,[162] cells appearing to be tetraploid comprised 5 to 10 per cent of total cells in fresh amnion specimens (not subjected to tissue culture). A similar proportion of tetraploid cells was noted in the short-term cultures that followed. Although in culture one cell line may outgrow another,[163] there was no evidence of preferential growth of the tetraploid cells in relation to the diploid cells or vice versa.[162] Of clinical consequence in this regard is the fact that only one case of tetraploidy has been described in a living infant with multiple congenital

Table 1 (Concluded).

| Location of Enzyme or Other Feature | Location of Enzyme Deficiency or Other Abnormality | Prenatal Diagnosis |
|---|---|---|
| None present | Cultured skin fibroblast | Potentially possible in future |
| Cultured skin fibroblast | Cultured skin fibroblast | Potentially possible in future |
| Cultured skin fibroblast | Unknown | Potentially possible in future |
| Cultured skin fibroblast | Cultured skin fibroblast | Potentially possible in future |
| Cultured skin fibroblast; cultured amniotic-fluid cell. | Cultured skin fibroblast; cultured amniotic-fluid cell. | Made |
| Cultured skin fibroblast; cultured amniotic-fluid cell. | Cultured skin fibroblast; cultured amniotic-fluid cell. | Made |
| Cultured skin fibroblast | Unknown | Potentially possible in future |
| Cultured skin fibroblast; amniotic fluid | Cultured skin fibroblast | Potentially possible in future |
| Cultured skin fibroblast; cultured amniotic-fluid cell. | | Possible |

189

anomalies who survived for 36 weeks.[164] Although tetraploid/diploid mosaicism was seen in the hematopoietic and lymphatic cells in this patient, fibroblast cultures derived from skin and other tissues were diploid. Tetraploidy has been noted, however, in abortuses.[165,166] Hughes and Csermely found that the endometrium is normally heteroploid, being partially composed of cells with aneuploid chromosome numbers.[167] Others, however, have failed to confirm these observations and report karyotypically normal diploid cells.[162]

In line with the recommendations of Court Brown et al.[168] for other tissues, it seems prudent in demonstrating the fetal karyotype to count at least 30 metaphases of the cultured amniotic-fluid cells. The possibility of mosaicism in the fetus may occasionally prove difficult to resolve. It has been emphasized, however, that a statistical approach is only a helpful guide and can never in itself prove the existence of mosaicism.[168]

The numerically most important indication for amniocentesis has become, and will probably remain, the prenatal diagnosis of chromosomal abnormality. Clearly, the high risks of bearing a chromosomally abnormal child, which we calculate to be about 1:40 between 40 and 44 years of age, provide cogent reasons for routine diagnostic amniocentesis in women over 40 years of age. When and if the procedure could be shown to have virtually no risk, a strong case could be made for routine amniocenteses in all pregnancies, based on the 1:200 chance of bearing a child with a significant chromosomal abnormality.[143]

When either parent is a known translocation carrier, or when familial nondisjunction is otherwise evident, the high risk of bearing a chromosomally abnormal child makes amniocentesis mandatory. This is one of the most clear-cut situations in which amniocentesis can be helpful in reassuring parents that the fetus is not affected, and has led us to search actively for such familial translocation carriers to counsel them. In more unusual carrier states, in which the chromosomes in question cannot be identified with certainty, it may not be possible to distinguish an abnormal from a normal karyotype definitively, and amniocentesis will therefore not be helpful in this situation.

A special problem arises for the family who already have a child with trisomy 21. There is some evidence of an increased risk for recurrence of trisomy 21.[149,169,170] However, until the exact risks are known, it remains extremely difficult to reassure a mother who has previously borne a child with mongolism. The management of these cases revolves around the informed consideration of the balance of risks for amniocentesis and subsequent abortion if necessary, the maternal age and the degree of maternal apprehension and depression.

Cytogenetic or chemical study of the abortus and amniotic fluid must be considered essential in each case, not only for the medicolegal reasons of confirming the diagnosis but also for the continuing rigorous quality control of the tests employed for prenatal studies.

## THE X-LINKED DISORDERS

The management of pregnant mothers who are carriers of X-linked disorders depends upon the sex of the fetus. Since fetal sex can be accurately determined in known maternal carriers, all male fetuses could be aborted. This approach, however, would result in the abortion of a normal male fetus in half the cases. A more rational way would be to make the specific prenatal diagnosis of an affected male. In the more common serious X-linked disorders (hemophilia, Duchenne muscular dystrophy and nephrogenic diabetes insipidus), a specific prenatal diagnosis is not possible at present. Both the Hunter and the Lesch–Nyhan syndromes, which are sex-linked disorders, can be specifically diagnosed in utero. Cultured skin fibroblasts from patients with the Lesch–Nyhan syndrome (X-linked hyperuricemia) have been shown to be deficient in hypoxanthine-guanine phosphoribosyltransferase activity.[171] With the use of autoradiographic methods and radioactive hypoxanthine, the affected cells fail to incorporate hypoxanthine and are seen to remain unlabeled. When this technic is applied to cultured amniotic-fluid cells, a set of identical twins, both with the Lesch–Nyhan syndrome, has been diagnosed in utero by DeMars et al.[172] Heterozygotes for this disorder have also been identified by the presence of two populations of equal numbers of enzyme-deficient and normal cells in the culture.[173]

Recently, factor-VIII-like activity has been demonstrated in normal and hemophilic cultured skin fibroblasts,[174] and if these observations are confirmed, the prenatal diagnosis of hemophilia may be possible. Certain characteristic features of Fabry's disease are evident in the leukocytes and cultured skin fibroblasts of these patients. This disorder is now potentially diagnosable in utero.

Different views can be expected on the question of abortion for a treatable, but presently incurable, disorder such as hemophilia or nephrogenic diabetes insipidus. This remains a parental decision based on the informed counsel of their physician.

## THE METABOLIC DISORDERS

Fundamental to progress in this group of disorders have been the observations that cultured skin fibroblasts retain their enzymatic machinery through successive generations in culture, thereby facilitating the demonstration of diminished or absent enzyme activity or the detection of excess storage material.

The prenatal diagnosis of certain inborn errors of metabolism by assay of the enzyme activity in cells cultured from amniotic fluid rests on the premise that cultured cells derived from skin accurately reflect the specific characteristics of the disorder under study. To an important degree, this premise seems to hold true. The manifestations of the inborn errors of metabolism that may be evident prenatally will be considered in cultured amniotic cells, noncultured amniotic cells and in amniotic fluid itself. Table 1 reflects this approach and also relates observations on cultured skin fibroblasts to those in amniotic cells or fluid, and to other tissues. Many of the disorders listed in Table 1 are not discussed in the text.

Usually, a family history of a disease in this group is obtained only if a previous child was affected. When a family history is indeed positive for a particular metabolic disorder it may well be possible to determine, for example, if either or both of the newly married couple are carriers. The demonstration that both parents are carriers for a particular disease evident in tissue culture could logically be followed by monitoring every pregnancy in this family, thereby preventing the birth of *any* affected offspring. In the second part of this paper the metabolic disorders will be discussed under the broad headings of diseases of lipid metabolism, the mucopolysaccharidoses, the amino acid and related disorders, disorders of carbohydrate metabolism, and an important miscellaneous group.

## DISORDERS OF LIPID METABOLISM

Sphingolipids are major components of all cell membranes and of particular importance to neural structure and function. In several well defined clinical disorders (Table 1), recently reviewed by Brady,[175] the accumulation of excessive quantities of particular sphingolipids can be demonstrated together with deficiencies of their respective sphingolipid hydrolases.

### Niemann–Pick Disease

Holtz et al.,[71] in 1964, by using quantitative thin-layer chromatography, first demonstrated that cultured fibroblasts from patients with Niemann–Pick disease accumulate almost twice as much sphingomyelin as control cells do. At the same time, they showed that fibroblasts derived from the amnion of an infant subsequently diagnosed as having Niemann–Pick disease also accumulated sphingomyelin in excess. This observation set the stage for the prenatal diagnosis of the lipid-storage diseases in general, and Niemann–Pick disease in particular.

The demonstration of deficient activity of a sphingomyelin-cleaving enzyme was observed in skin fibroblast cultures derived from patients with two forms of Niemann–Pick disease.[73] Sphingomyelinase activity in cultured amniotic-fluid fibroblasts has been demonstrated,[175] and it may now be possible to diagnose Niemann–Pick disease in utero. Heterozygous carriers have not as yet been detected by enzyme assays of skin or amniotic-fluid fibroblasts.

Cultured fibroblasts from bone marrow and skin from patients with Crocker's Types[176] A, B and D of Niemann–Pick disease were examined for sphingomyelinase activities.[74] Types A and D had very low levels of enzyme activity, so that theoretically it should be possible to diagnose both prenatally. The prenatal diagnosis of Type D, however, does not appear possible at present because the activity of sphingomyelinase in cultured fibroblasts was similar to controls.

## Gaucher's Disease

In this disease the lipid glucocerebroside accumulates in spleen, liver and bone marrow. The biochemical defect is now taken to be a deficiency of the enzyme that hydrolyzes glucocerebroside.[51,52] Glucocerebrosidase activity is normally demonstrable in cultured skin fibroblasts, and in one patient with infantile Gaucher's disease this enzyme activity was almost completely absent.[175] Intermediate levels of glucocerebrosidase activity in fibroblast cultures were obtained from heterozygous carriers of Gaucher's disease.[175] Amniotic-fluid fibroblasts in culture also contain glucocerebrosidase activity so that the diagnosis of Gaucher's disease in utero is now possible.

## Metachromatic Leukodystrophy

This degenerative brain disease is characterized by the accumulation of an acidic sphingoglycolipid called sulfatide in neural tissue, kidney and bile ducts.[50] Patients with this disease excrete increased quantities of sulfatide in the urine. The biochemical defect has been shown to be a deficiency of a sulfuric acid esterase.[177,178] This observation has been used to explain the resulting accumulation of sulfatide principally within the central nervous system. At least three arylsulfatases (A, B and C) are present in mammalian tissues, which can be conveniently detected by measurement of the hydrolysis of artificial substrates, such as p-nitrocatechol sulfate.[66] In patients with classic metachromatic leukodystrophy both arylsulfatase A and cerebroside sulfatase activity have been shown to be deficient.[67] The activity of arylsulfatase A is diminished in both urine[179] and leukocytes[180] in these patients. In a less common variant arylsulfatases A, B and C as well as steroid sulfatase are deficient.[68,180]

Skin fibroblasts from patients with metachromatic leukodystrophy have been shown to have markedly decreased levels of arylsulfatase A activities.[69,70] Arylsulfatase A activity has also been detected in cultured amniotic-fluid fibroblasts.[70] A deficiency of this lysosomal enzyme in cultured cells has allowed the prenatal diagnosis of metachromatic leukodystrophy in one case.[28] The detection of the heterozygote for the disease is now possible on the basis of arylsulfatase A activities in cultured skin fibroblasts.[70]

The level of arylsulfatase A activity in normal cultured amniotic-fluid cells is lower than in normal skin cells. Since heterozygote amniotic cells might be anticipated to have quite low enzyme activity, it may prove difficult to differentiate the heterozygote from the affected fetus.[70]

### Fabry's Disease

Affected males with this sex-linked disorder generally die in the third or fourth decade of life from renal failure.[50] A sphingoglycolipid, ceramide trihexoside, accumulates in the tissues and cultured skin fibroblasts of these patients.[47,48,181] The metabolic defect in this disease has been shown to be a deficiency of an enzyme that catalyzes the hydrolysis of the terminal molecule of galactose of ceramide trihexoside.[47] In addition to glycolipid accumulation in skin fibroblasts in this disorder, a markedly elevated acid mucopolysaccharide content has been found.[48] Female carriers of this disease show intermediate levels of hydrolytic activity in their tissues. Recently, alpha-galactosidase activity was found to be deficient in the leukocytes of patients with Fabry's disease.[49] Observations by Sweeley have indicated a deficiency of ceramide trihexoside hydrolysis in plasma from patients with Fabry's disease.[182] No differences in p-nitrophenol galactoside hydrolysis were noted. It seems probable that by the use of synthetic substrates for the enzyme assays, the prenatal diagnosis of Fabry's disease will be achieved.

### Globoid Leukodystrophy (Krabbe's Disease)

This is a fatal demyelinating disease characterized by progressive neurologic deterioration beginning between the third and fifth months of life, with death before one year.[181] Austin reported a relative increase of ceramide galactoside and a decrease of sulfatide so that total glycolipid is not markedly changed,[183] but the ratio of cerebroside to sulfatide is increased. He and his co-workers also found a deficiency of cerebroside sulfating enzyme,[184] but the enzyme system responsible for this reaction has not yet been fully evaluated. Independently, Eto and Suzuki[185] and Malone[186] have reported marked deficiency of galactocerebrosidase activity in brain tissue and in leukocytes from patients with Krabbe's disease. There seems to be every likelihood that, as

195

in the other sphingolipidoses, this disorder, which is evident in tissue culture, will become diagnosable in utero.

### Tay – Sachs Disease (G$_{M2}$ Gangliosidosis)

This heredodegenerative disorder of infancy becomes clinically manifest by about the fifth month of life. About one of 40 Ashkenazi Jews and about one of 380 non-Jewish persons are heterozygous for the gene of Tay–Sachs disease.[187] These gene frequencies correspond to 158 births of infants with Tay–Sachs disease per 1,000,000 among the Ashkenazi Jews and 1.7 per 1,000,000 among non-Jews.[188]

In this disease G$_{M2}$ ganglioside and to a lesser extent its asialoceramide trihexoside derivative[53] are stored in the central nervous system. Smaller accumulations of G$_{M2}$ ganglioside have been found in other tissues as well,[59] including cultured skin fibroblasts.[60] The G$_{M2}$ ganglioside storage appears to result from a block in the catabolism of the sphingolipid that is due to the absence of a specific hexosaminidase (hexosaminidase A). This enzyme can be demonstrated in extracts from frozen organs, plasma and serum, leukocytes and cultured fibroblasts.[61,62,189] Kolodny et al.[60] were able to diagnose Tay–Sachs disease in a six-week-old child because of a substantial increase in the level of G$_{M2}$ ganglioside in a cell line cultured from the umbilical cord of this child at birth. Recently, Schneck et al.[63] reported a case of Tay–Sachs disease diagnosed during the second trimester of pregnancy. They demonstrated in this case a virtual absence of hexosaminidase A activity in the amniotic fluid and the uncultured amniotic-fluid cells, and subsequently showed enzyme deficiency in the liver and brain of the abortus. Earlier observations by these authors[63] on cultured tissue of an eight-week-old embryo from a mother heterozygous for Tay–Sachs disease indicated that the fetal deficiency of hexosaminidase A in conjunction with G$_{M2}$ accumulation is detectable very early in gestation.

Differentiation of the heterozygous carrier from the homozygote with Tay–Sachs disease is possible with the serum assay of O'Brien et al.[64] If complete accuracy in the prenatal diagnosis of this disease is to be achieved, it will be necessary to demonstrate a similar clear-cut differentiation in utero between the heterozygote and the affected homozygote.

Clinically indistinguishable from the classic form of Tay–Sachs disease is a disorder seen thus far only in non-Jews that is characterized by excess storage of $G_{M2}$ ganglioside and its asialo derivative in the central nervous system and of globoside in visceral organs.[54,65] Enzyme preparations from brain, liver, kidneys[54,65] and cultured skin fibroblasts of patients with this disease are almost totally deficient in hexosaminidase (hexosaminidase A and B) activity.

Accurate diagnosis of Tay–Sachs disease requires determinations of both the total amount of hexosaminidase and the ratio of hexosaminidase A to hexosaminidase B, because although very low levels of total hexosaminidase activity characterize the unusual form of Tay–Sachs disease, the ratio of the residual hexosaminidase A to B activity is normal. In the more common form of the disease, hexosaminidase A activity is low or absent, but the residual hexosaminidase activity is normal or elevated owing to a greater than normal amount of hexosaminidase B activity. Therefore, as with other inborn metabolic errors, to simplify the prenatal diagnosis of the Tay–Sachs group of diseases, careful studies, when possible, of the genotype of both parents and of any affected siblings should be undertaken before amniocentesis.

### $G_{M1}$ Gangliosidosis (Generalized Gangliosidosis)[55]

This rare storage disease is characterized by the neuronal accumulation of $G_{M1}$ ganglioside and its sialic acid-free parent compound ceramide tetrahexoside and, in addition, the visceral accumulation of a highly water-soluble undersulfated mucopolysaccharide of the keratan-sulfate type with a related, less soluble sialomucopolysaccharide.[56] Only 20 cases are on record.[55,190]

A deficiency of the enzyme β-galactosidase would best explain the accumulation of these otherwise unrelated substances in this disease. This was first demonstrated by Sacrez and Hers[191] on a liver-biopsy specimen with the use of an artificial substrate. Subsequently, others found deficient β-galactosidase activity in a wide variety of tissues, including brain, liver, spleen, kidney, leukocytes and cultured skin fibroblasts.[55,57,190,192,193]

So far as the visceral mucopolysaccharide storage

is concerned, Wolfe et al.[190] have found that the urine of one patient contained greatly increased amounts of undersulfated keratan-sulfate-type mucopolysaccharides. Deficient $\beta$-galactosidase activity has also been noted in the urine of these patients.[55] Amniotic fluid per se has not as yet been examined for $\beta$-galactosidase activity or the excessive accumulation of a specific undersulfated keratan-sulfate type of mucopolysaccharide.

Sloan et al.,[57] having detected a specific deficiency of $G_{M1}$-$\beta$-galactosidase in cultured skin fibroblasts, have also developed a simple histochemical test for $\beta$-galactosidase. Fibroblasts grown on cover slips are incubated with 5-bromo-4-chloro-3-indolyl-$\beta$-D-galactopyranoside. The control cells stain indigo blue owing to the liberation of the aglycone indicating the presence of normal $\beta$-galactosidase activity whereas the patient's cells remain colorless[58] since the substrate is not cleaved.

Extension of these and similar technics to cultured amniotic-fluid cells can be expected to facilitate the early intrauterine diagnosis of $G_{M1}$-gangliosidosis. This is especially likely since the types and relative amounts of ganglioside[60] and the activity of $\beta$-galactosidase in cultured skin and amniotic-fluid fibroblasts[57] are nearly identical.

Caution should be exercised in the biochemical differentiation of $G_{M1}$-gangliosidosis from the Hurler–Hunter syndrome. In both diseases gangliosides and mucopolysaccharides accumulate, and $\beta$-galactosidase activity is depressed. However, the reduction in $\beta$-galactosidase activity is not quantitatively as great in the Hurler–Hunter syndrome.[78] Furthermore, starch-gel electrophoresis of the various $\beta$-galactosidase components gives different and characteristic results for these disorders. Ho and O'Brien[79] have reported that the slow moving components of $\beta$-galactosidase from liver tissue of patients with Hurler's syndrome were markedly deficient. In $G_{M1}$-gangliosidosis, both the slow moving components and the fast moving components of $\beta$-galactosidase were greatly reduced.[79]

It should be possible to make an intrauterine diagnosis of $G_{M1}$-gangliosidosis through the demonstration in cultured amniotic-fluid cells of a low level of $\beta$-galactosidase activity coupled with the near absence of both the slow and fast moving components of this enzyme. Accumulation of $G_{M1}$-

ganglioside and of specific mucopolysaccharides within these cells would provide additional support for this diagnosis. Thomas[194] has also shown a $\beta$-D-galactosidase deficiency in the urine of a patient with generalized gangliosidosis. Therefore, the prenatal diagnosis of $G_{M1}$-gangliosidosis seems possible if either the amniotic cells or the fluid of an affected fetus (or both) can be shown to be specifically deficient in the activity of this enzyme.

Generalized gangliosidosis and Tay–Sachs disease are only two of the five or more recognized gangliosidoses. Other diseases of ganglioside storage have been proposed,[195] but since they are confined to single case reports and have not been studied enzymatically, they will not be considered in this review.

### Refsum's Disease (Heredopathia Atactica Polyneuritiformis)

In this hereditary storage disease large amounts of an unusual fatty acid, phytanic acid, accumulate in all body tissues.[75] The pathway for the metabolism of phytanic acid has been delineated in some elegant experiments on cultured skin fibroblasts.[76] Heterozygotes can now be distinguished since they appear to oxidize phytanic acid at approximately half the rate of normal controls. Since cultured amniotic cells have been shown to have the capacity to oxidize phytanic acid,[77] the prenatal diagnosis of Refsum's disease has become a possibility.

### THE MUCOPOLYSACCHARIDOSES

In this group of disorders certain mucopolysaccharides accumulate in the tissues, the urine and in cultured skin fibroblasts. McKusick[80] has separated six entities on the basis of their clinical features, their mode of inheritance and the nature of the accumulated mucopolysaccharide. Almost certainly several additional types exist.[196] The prenatal diagnosis of the mucopolysaccharide disorders is now feasible through study of cultured amniotic-fluid cells and of the amniotic fluid itself.

### Cultured-Fibroblast Studies

The production of mucopolysaccharides in tissue culture has been known for many years.[197-199] Evidence that Hurler's syndrome was manifest in cultured skin fibroblasts was first presented by Danes

199

and Bearn.[200] They employed histochemical technics for demonstrating metachromasia in cultured fibroblasts in this disease. The nonspecific nature of metachromasia in cultured skin or amniotic-fluid fibroblasts[201] has prevented its use alone for the prenatal diagnosis of mucopolysaccharidoses or other disorders.

The quantitative estimation of mucopolysaccharide production by cultured fibroblasts could provide an important prenatal diagnostic tool. Cultured skin fibroblasts derived from normal persons synthesize a variety of sulfated mucopolysaccharides, including dermatan sulfate.[202] Danes and Bearn[81] reported increased mucopolysaccharide accumulation in cultured skin fibroblasts in Hurler's syndrome, and indicated that this technic could be used to distinguish the affected person and the carrier from the normal subject. Recently, a striking increase of dermatan sulfate in cultured skin fibroblasts in the syndromes of Hurler, Hunter and Sanfilippo, and late infantile amaurotic familial idiocy[203] has been reported.

Thus far, neither heparitin sulfate nor keratan sulfate has been found in skin fibroblasts from any of the patients with the mucopolysaccharidoses,[82,203] and it is not known whether these cells synthesize these polysaccharides. Although Sanfilippo's syndrome is characterized by the excretion of heparitin sulfate in urine, cultured skin fibroblasts in this disorder store dermatan sulfate.[82] In contrast skin fibroblasts in Morquio's disease appear to have an increased amount, but normal distribution of acid mucopolysaccharides.[82] Whereas cultured amniotic-fluid cells have not been studied for mucopolysaccharide accumulation by quantitative chemical analysis, the inability to grow sufficient cells in the short time available unfortunately places severe limitations on prospects of using this method for the prenatal diagnosis of the mucopolysaccharidoses. The advent of microcolumn technics, already in use for quantitative mucopolysaccharide estimation,[204,205] however, may prove useful in this regard.

The enzymatic basis of the mucopolysaccharidoses is not yet known. However, Van Hoof and Hers[206] and others[79] have described a deficiency of a specific β-galactosidase isoenzyme in liver and kidney tissues of patients with Hurler's syndrome. The diminished β-galactosidase activity may be secondary to the polysaccharide accumulation. Neither cultured skin nor amniotic cells in the mucopolysaccharidoses have yet been reported to have deficient galactosidase activity.

Fratantoni et al.[83] have successfully employed radioactive sulfate ($^{35}SO_4$) incorporation as a diagnostic tool in the Hurler and Hunter syndromes. Their earlier studies on cultured skin fibroblasts from patients with these disorders showed that the cells of affected persons accumulate $^{35}SO_4$-labeled mucopolysaccharide at a linear rate, whereas normal cells reach a steady state within two days.[207] Cells from heterozygotes display an essentially normal pattern. Amniotic cells obtained from a pregnant known heterozygous mother showed abnormal kinetics of $^{35}SO_4$ incorporation identical to those of the fibroblasts from an affected sibling, and easily distinguishable from normal amniotic-fluid cell controls and the skin fibroblasts of the parents. The outcome of this pregnancy was a female infant with Hurler's syndrome. In a further case studied in the same way the prenatal diagnosis of Hunter's syndrome was made, but attempts at confirmation on the macerated abortus were unsuccessful.[83]

This technic holds great promise as a reliable prenatal diagnostic tool. Improved methods for culturing amniotic-fluid cells will be necessary to provide timely results. Further studies will be required to establish clearly the normal, as well as heterozygous, ranges for $^{35}SO_4$ incorporation and the variables involved (cell confluency, duration in culture and so forth). No information is yet available on $^{35}SO_4$ incorporation into mucopolysaccharide in amniotic-fluid cells in the mucopolysaccharidoses or other disorders in which intracellular mucopolysaccharide accumulation is increased.

Fratantoni et al.,[208] again using $^{35}SO_4$, have devised another test, to make the prenatal diagnosis of Hurler's or Hunter's syndrome. It is based on their observation that cells of different genotypes, when mixed in culture, interact to give kinetic patterns of $^{35}SO_4$ incorporation that are within normal limits, whereas cells of the same genotype do not. Their studies suggest that some factor (or factors) (probably protein) enters one cell line (for example, from Hurler's syndrome) from another (such as a normal person) and remedies the block in the degradative pathway for mucopolysaccharides. The reason why, in Hunter heterozygotes (actually mosaics of normal and Hunter cells), the cells without the mutant gene do not correct the affected cells[85] requires further investigation.

In Hurler's syndrome ascorbic acid is known not only to increase the synthesis of sulfated mucopolysaccharides in fibroblast cell cultures, but also to produce selective retention of these mucopolysaccharides within the cell.[209,210] Introduction of vitamin A alcohol — in contrast to ascorbic acid — into fibroblast cultures in Hunter's syndrome results in both an intracellular and an extracellular reduction of about 60 per cent in total mucopolysaccharide content.[211] The total mucopolysaccharide content in normal fibroblast cultures is reduced by about 30 per cent. The effects of both ascorbic acid and vitamin A on cultured amniotic-fluid cells from normal and affected fetuses are unknown at present, but may ultimately prove useful for intrauterine diagnostic tests.

### Amniotic-Fluid Studies

Recently, the presence of dermatan sulfate has been demonstrated in normal amniotic fluid, whereas heparitin sulfate was not detected. Matalon and Dorfman,[84] in applying their observations, have been able to diagnose Hurler's syndrome in utero by demonstrating excessive amounts of dermatan sulfate and the presence of heparitin sulfate in the amniotic fluid. Since the fetal urine is the most likely source of these mucopolysaccharides, it should be possible to diagnose all the mucopolysaccharidoses in which dermatan sulfate, heparitin sulfate and possibly even keratan sulfate are excreted in the fetal urine. Since cultured fibroblasts in Morquio's syndrome do not produce keratan sulfate (which the patients with the syndrome do excrete in their urine), quantitative chemical analysis of amniotic fluid should prove diagnostic if indeed the urine of the affected fetus does contain this mucopolysaccharide.

Danes et al.[212] have indicated that the mucopolysaccharide content of the amniotic fluid is relatively high early in gestation, and thereafter decreases steadily until term. They suggest that serial amniocentesis might be helpful in prenatal diagnosis, since the mucopolysaccharide content of the amniotic fluid normally shows a steady decrease throughout gestation, whereas fluid from an affected fetus would be expected to have a persistently elevated mucopolysaccharide content throughout gestation.

Not unexpectedly, many variables operate to influence mucopolysaccharide production in cell culture, and include growth rate, cell density, cell age and composition of the culture medium.[213] For example, stimulation of mucopolysaccharide synthesis by embryo extract may occur.[214] A concentration of 5 per cent serum may give optimum production of hyaluronic acid by rat-skin fibroblasts, whereas concentrations above 10 per cent may cause marked inhibition of mucopolysaccharide synthesis.[215] These workers also showed that trypsinization of fibroblast monolayers may release considerable amounts of hyaluronic acid, which is presumably bound to the cell surface.[213]

Until the enzymatic basis of the mucopolysaccharidoses is known, prenatal diagnoses in this group will depend upon $^{35}SO_4$ incorporation by cultured amniotic-fluid cells and quantitative chemical analysis for mucopolysaccharides in the amniotic fluid itself. It would perhaps be most reliable at present to employ both technics for prenatal diagnosis in this group.

### THE AMINO ACID DISORDERS

The frequency of the detectable amino acid disorders is approximately 1:3000 live births.[216] Although some of these disorders are associated with severe illness, mental retardation or early death, a few cause no symptoms, have only minor clinical manifestations or are treatable to a greater or lesser degree. The decision to establish a prenatal diagnosis in this group must take into account the nature of the disorder, as well as the risk of amniocentesis and the wishes of the parents. The prenatal diagnosis of the genetic amino-acid disorders will be approached by examination of the cultured amniotic-fluid cells, the noncultured amniotic-fluid cells and the amniotic fluid itself.

#### Cultured Amniotic-Fluid Cells

An increasing number of enzymes have been shown to be active in cultured amniotic-fluid cells, and therefore are potentially useful for the prenatal diagnosis of specific disorders (see Table 1). Owing to the rarity of these disorders, opportunities to study carrier mothers have been limited. Amniocenteses have been performed on expectant mothers who were known heterozygotes for both homocystinuria[92] (cystathionine synthase deficiency) and maple-syrup-urine disease in three cases[11,99] (branched-chain keto acid decarboxylase deficiency). Fetal cells cultured from the amniotic fluid in two of these cases contained normal levels of the corresponding enzyme in question. Both infants were healthy after delivery and had no evidence of disease. The amniotic cells in the third case showed deficient enzyme activity, and the infant at birth had maple-syrup-urine disease.[99]

**Noncultured Amniotic-Fluid Cells**

A second line of approach is the measurement of enzymes in noncultured amniotic-fluid cells. Recently, Nadler[93] investigated the enzyme contents of such cells by measuring enzyme activities in the cells sedimented from 2 to 10 ml of amniotic fluid. The enzymes shown to be present in these cells were also detected in cultivated amniotic-fluid cells (Table 1). Enzyme activity was highest in the cells that were obtained before 20 weeks of gestation. No or low activity of the enzymes was detected in cells obtained after this period, confirming an earlier observation made by Dancis.[18]

It is interesting that ornithine carbamyltransferase activity thought to be absent in cultured cells has now been detected in noncultured amniotic-fluid cells.[93] This would make possible the antenatal diagnosis of hyper-ammonemia Type II (ornithine carbamyltransferase deficiency), a disorder usually associated with mental retardation. Phenylalanine hydroxylase and histidase activities have not been demonstrated in cells cultured in vitro.[217] Therefore, enzymatic diagnosis of phenylketonuria and histidinemia cannot at present be made by tissue-culture technics. But for several other disorders the direct assay of enzyme activity in noncultured cells may be a rapid, economic and simple screening or diagnostic technic.

**Amniotic Fluid**

Thirdly, since amniotic fluid is derived partly from fetal urine, direct analysis for chemicals that reflect metabolic or transport disorders could provide a rapid quantitative method for prenatal diagnosis. In a preliminary study, Levy et al.[218] have studied the normal values for free amino acids in amniotic fluid between 14 and 18 weeks' gestation. The relative concentrations of the free amino acids were similar in the amniotic-fluid samples studied. Some specimens tended to have greater concentrations of all amino acids than others, a variation apparently independent of gestational age and creatinine concentration.

At 14 to 18 weeks' gestation the quantities of many of the free amino acids in amniotic fluid appeared to be different to those at term.[219] Those amino acids, more concentrated in the amniotic fluid at 14 to 18 weeks, include valine, methionine, leucine, phenylalanine, tyrosine, lysine, histidine, arginine, proline and glutamic acid, whereas lesser concentrations of taurine, aspartic acid, serine and glutamine were found.[218]

Opportunities have not been available to test whether disorders of renal amino acid transport such as Hartnup disease (defect of neutral amino acid transport) and cystinuria might be demonstrated by the finding of an increased amount of the specific group of amino acids in the amniotic fluid.[220] The placental circulation, however, may easily be able to remove any accumulating metabolites in the amniotic fluid, as exemplified by the normal amino acid pattern of the umbilical-cord blood at birth of infants with phenylketonuria. Therefore, the presence of easily measurable quantities of phenylalanine in the amniotic fluid at 14 to 18 weeks of gestation, even if fetal in origin, is also unlikely to prove useful for diagnostic purposes.

### DISORDERS OF CARBOHYDRATE METABOLISM

In cultured cells the metabolism of glucose proceeds by way of the Embden–Meyerhof pathway, as in the tissues of the living organism. Cultured cells have also been shown to possess the capacity to synthesize glycogen.[221]

### FUCOSIDOSIS

This profound progressive cerebral degenerative disorder,[104] in which excessive storage of fucose occurs, is associated with alpha-fucosidase deficiency.[105] Activity of this enzyme is detectable in cultured amniotic-fluid cells and renders this dis-

205

order diagnosable before birth.[106]

## GALACTOSEMIA

This disorder, which is a hereditary inborn error in the metabolism of galactose due to galactose-1-P uridyltransferase deficiency, was first demonstrated to be evident in tissue culture by Krooth and Weinberg.[112] Since cultured amniotic-fluid cells have been shown to have galactose-1-P uridyltransferase activity, the prenatal diagnosis of galactosemia is now possible. A known maternal heterozygote, who had previously given birth to a galactosemic child, had an amniocentesis before elective cesarean section at 33 weeks' gestation. The cultured fetal cells contained no detectable galactose-1-P uridyltransferase activity. The diagnosis was confirmed by the demonstration that this enzyme activity was absent in the cord blood of the infant.[113]

## GLYCOGEN-STORAGE DISEASES

In patients with Type II glycogenosis (Pompe's disease) alpha-1, 4-glucosidase activity is deficient in the liver,[50] leukocytes and cultured fibroblasts.[107,108] This enzyme has also been demonstrated in cultivated and noncultivated amniotic-fluid cells.[109] Nadler and Messina[109] and Cox et al.[110] have reported the prenatal diagnosis of this disease in three cases. They demonstrated a deficiency of alpha-1, 4-glucosidase activity in cultured amniotic-fluid cells from known maternal heterozygotes. Alpha-1, 4-glucosidase is present in normal amniotic fluid, which can therefore be assayed directly for diagnostic purposes. Cox et al.[110] pointed out that in this disorder, bloody contamination of amniotic fluid could be dealt with by centrifugation of all cellular elements and the supernatant fluid analyzed for alpha-1, 4-glucosidase activity.

In Type IV glycogenosis (amylopectinosis), which is the rarest of the glycogen-storage diseases, there is a deficiency of debrancher enzyme demonstrable in the liver and cultured skin fibroblasts.[50,111] Howell et al.[111] have shown that this enzyme is active in cultured amniotic-fluid cells, making the antenatal diagnosis of this fatal disease possible.

Type III glycogenosis[50] has recently been characterized in cultured skin fibroblasts by demonstration of the amylo-1, 6-glucosidase deficiency.[11] The presence of this enzyme in normal amniotic-fluid cells[11] should allow the prenatal diagnosis of this disorder. The other three types of glycogen-storage disease have not as yet been demonstrated in tissue culture.

## MANNOSIDOSIS

Affected patients clinically resemble those with Hurler's syndrome, but accumulate excessive amounts of mannose and glucosamine.[115] Biochemical studies of the liver have revealed an alpha-mannosidase deficiency.[116] Since alpha-mannosidase activity is detectable in cultured amniotic-fluid cells,[106] it appears that mannosidosis may be diagnosed in utero.

## MISCELLANEOUS DISORDERS

### Adrenogenital Syndrome

This autosomal recessive disorder is due to defects in the biosynthesis of the adrenocorticosteroids. The syndrome has been diagnosed before birth in four infants by the demonstration of greater than normal amounts of 17-ketosteroids and pregnanetriol in the amniotic fluid at term, or by increased maternal urinary estriol.[121,122-124] In one infant antenatal therapy was attempted during the 39th week of pregnancy, and serial intrauterine injection of cortisone resulted in a fall in the pregnanetriol content in the amniotic fluid. A study by Merkatz et al.[125] was at variance with these reports. They showed that the steroid concentration in the amniotic fluid at term in an affected infant was only slightly elevated, and concluded that its value in the diagnosis of the adrenogenital syndrome requires further investigation. Measurement of the steroids during the first two trimesters of pregnancy did not help to distinguish between an affected and an unaffected fetus.

### Congenital Malformations

Spectrophotometric examination of amniotic fluid is extensively used to provide an index of the severity of erythroblastosis affecting the fetus in Rh-sensitized pregnancies. Amniotic fluids possessing absorption spectra similar to those seen in severely affected Rh-sensitized pregnancies have been found in association with at least seven cases of anencephaly,[222] one with duodenal atresia[223] and another with craniosynostosis, polysyndactyly and pyloric stenosis.[224] All these cases were *not* associated with

207

Rh disease, and the origin of this chromogen remains obscure. Clinical application of this technic to the intrauterine diagnosis of congenital malformations in general is not advised at present, pending further study of the origin and effects of this chromogen. Of interest are the studies by Nelson[225] of amniotic fluid derived from several abnormal pregnancies (prematurity, respiratory-distress syndrome and anencephaly with polyhydramnios) that showed low total lipid, low total phospholipid and a decreased percentage of lecithin in the phospholipid fraction.

Examination of the fetus with a fiberoptic instrument is already possible.[11] The use of ultrasound,[31,32] already referred to for placental localization, could readily be used for the determination of head size. By the 14th week the fetal head is definitely recognizable,[33] making it theoretically possible to diagnose hydrocephalus or microcephaly (if already manifest) before 24 weeks' gestation. The establishment of normal variations in fetal-head size in relation to body size should precede any diagnostic efforts in this regard. Fetal growth retardation or even overgrowth may also be detectable by this method.

The teratogenic or other harmful effects on the fetus from drugs ingested by the mother or from viral infection in utero present future opportunities for prenatal diagnosis. Whereas LSD and other drugs may be associated with chromosomal breakage or other abnormalities,[226] these are usually nonspecific. The presence or importance of an infectious agent or its associated antibodies (for example, cytomegalovirus and toxoplasmosis) in amniotic cells or fluid will require further study. These disorders of "environmental" origin cannot as yet be reliably diagnosed in utero. The use of amniography, however, may prove useful for the detection of congenital malformations[227] in selected pregnancies (for example, polyhydramnios).

### Congenital Erythropoietic Porphyria

This has recently been shown to be evident in cultured skin fibroblasts.[127] These cells in porphyric patients have a lower specific activity of cosynthetase than in normal controls, the heterozygote values being intermediate. Although the prenatal diagnosis may eventually be made by means of cultured amniotic-fluid cells, the possible presence of excessive amounts of uroporphyrin in the amniotic fluid itself requires evaluation.

## Cystic Fibrosis

Danes and Bearn first showed that cystic fibrosis was manifest in cultured skin fibroblasts.[128,129] The method employed demonstrated metachromasia in cultured skin fibroblasts after staining with toluidine blue. We have previously commented upon the nonspecific nature of this test,[201] and others have found a significant frequency of metachromasia in a random patient population.[228] Nadler[130] has also found that this technic is not reliable for prenatal diagnosis of cystic fibrosis. Electron microscopy of cultured skin fibroblasts in cystic fibrosis has not proved to be of any diagnostic help.[229] Recently, Gibbs has found decreased activity of $\beta$-glucuronidase in certain skin components in children with cystic fibrosis.[131] $\beta$-glucuronidase activity in tissue culture in cystic fibrosis has not yet been studied.

In quantitative and qualitative studies on cultured skin fibroblasts from patients with cystic fibrosis, an increase in the intracellular mucopolysaccharide content was observed, whereas the relative amounts of hyaluronic acid, dermatan sulfate and chondroitin sulfate were similar to those found in normal controls.[132] Others,[230] however, have found that no storage of mucopolysaccharides occurred within cultured fibroblasts of patients with cystic fibrosis, but rather that mucopolysaccharide accumulation was found extracellularly. Although technical or methodologic differences probably explain these contrasting results, no similar quantitative studies have yet been reported for amniotic-fluid fibroblasts. Recently, the glycogen content of fibroblasts was found to be increased in cystic fibrosis and other disorders,[231] suggesting that the accumulation of both glycogen and mucopolysaccharide in this disease may be nonspecific.

## I-cell Disease

Leroy and DeMars[133] studied cultured fibroblasts from patients with I-cell disease (so named because of the dark, cytoplasmic inclusions that surround the nucleus and juxtanuclear zone), who have a phenotype similar to Hurler's syndrome but without corneal clouding or excessive mucopolysacchariduria. Their fibroblasts were found to differ from normal controls and from patients with Hurler's syndrome not only in their abundant cytoplasmic inclusions, but also in the striking diminution of β-glucuronidase, and elevations in acid phosphatase.[134] The specificity of these findings requires further study. The prenatal diagnosis of I-cell disease has not as yet been made, but remains theoretically possible.

### Lysosomal Acid Phosphatase Deficiency

This new familial metabolic disorder is described by Nadler and Egan.[138] Acid phosphatase activity appears to be low in the lysosomal fraction of cultured fibroblasts, brain, liver, spleen and kidney in this disease. Nadler had previously demonstrated that acid phosphatase activity was detectable in cultured amniotic-fluid cells.[232] It has therefore been possible to make the prenatal diagnosis of this disorder in a patient of 13 weeks' gestation whose cultured amniotic-fluid cells were found to be deficient in acid phosphatase activity.[138]

### Marfan's Syndrome

This autosomal dominant disorder is manifest in cultured skin fibroblasts by the excessive production of hyaluronic acid.[139] No amniotic-fluid cell studies have yet been done, but since manifest in culture, this disorder becomes potentially diagnosable in utero.

### Myotonic Muscular Dystrophy

This autosomal dominant disorder with protean manifestations has recently been noted to be manifest in cultured skin fibroblasts.[233] These cells have been reported to exhibit marked metachromasia after staining with alcian blue, and to differ in their pattern of growth at a high density in culture. Confirmation of these observations and further biochemical definition could open the way for the prenatal diagnosis of a disorder that becomes clinically manifest usually in adulthood but occasionally in infancy.

### Xeroderma Pigmentosum

This disorder with skin manifestations is due to

the deficiency of an enzyme involved in the repair of DNA.[141] The presence of this "repair enzyme" in cultured amniotic-fluid cells makes the prenatal diagnosis possible.[142]

### Additional Disorders

It is important to realize that many additional disorders not shown in Table 1 are evident in tissue culture.[234,235] In this paper they are not considered appropriate for amniocentesis and subsequent abortion either because the criteria for diagnosis in culture are inadequate or the disease is mild in severity or late in onset. Gout,[236] diabetes mellitus,[237] progeria[238] and other disorders exemplify this group.

## TISSUE-CULTURE AND BIOCHEMICAL CONSIDERATIONS

Recent reviews on the genetic and biochemical aspects of cultured mammalian cells underscore the rapid advances in somatic cell genetics.[235,239-241] The prenatal diagnosis of increasing numbers of metabolic disorders has become a reality, and with it the need to have detailed knowledge of amniotic-fluid formation, kinetics, cellular components and chemical composition. Crucial to the informed interpretation of the rapidly accumulating prenatal studies is an understanding of certain characteristics of cultured cells, and some aspects of their biochemical functions and metabolic controls.

Divorced from hormonal and other influences operative in vivo, cultured cells differ in that they divide every 16 to 30 hours, in contrast to the generation time of 30 to 90 days in the living organism.[241] Human fibroblasts have a life-span of 50 to 70 generations in culture, and usually remain diploid until their terminal phases.[241] The 100-fold to 10,000-fold dilution that cells undergo when cultured from living tissue leads to the elution of materials that the cell can synthesize but must retain at metabolically effective levels to grow or function. Nevertheless, there has been no evidence that cells in tissues differ from cultured cells in their ability to transport and concentrate amino acids.[242]

There is an initial lag in the establishment of a culture, during which cellular adaptation to in vitro growth is occurring, and it may last a few hours to many days, depending upon many factors. Metabol-

ic activity during this period may be profoundly
affected, as reflected by a wide variety of enzyme
activities.[243]

The degree of cell confluency in culture may
affect enzyme activity. An increase in glucose-6-
phosphate dehydrogenase[243] and glucuronidase[244]
activities of cultured fibroblasts has been found
with densely confluent cultures. Moreover, cyclic
changes in lactic dehydrogenase activity in cell cultures may also occur.[243] Enzyme activity may vary
during the growth cycle of cells in culture.
Russell[114] has demonstrated that galactose-1-P-uridyl
transferase activity of both normal and galactosemic
cultured fibroblasts increased logarithmically during
growth. In normal cultures there was an increase of
2½ times in transferase activity per milligram of
protein from the time of subculture to the stage
when a dense cell population is maintained. The
mutant strain had negligible enzyme activity initially after subculture, but had low appreciable activity
after 160 hours of culture. Heterozygosity could easily be distinguished when cell cultures were compared at the same stage of growth; however, confu-
sion could arise if the properly timed comparison
were not made. It is possible that morphologically
different amniotic-fluid cells also differ in enzyme
activities. Thus far, Kaback,[11] in studying cultures
that were predominantly epithelioid, fibroblastic or
mixed, found no differences in the activities of hexosaminidase, β-galactosidase or arylsulfatase.

These points illustrate some possible difficulties
in the separation of heterozygous from the homozygous affected fetus and the importance of establishing normal variations. Of additional consequence
are the changes in enzyme activity that occur as
gestation proceeds. Glucose-6-$PO_4$ dehydrogenase
was found to be twice normal in the cells obtained
at 10 weeks' gestation, and an extra band was demonstrated by starch-gel electrophoresis.[232] Repeat
amniocentesis and subsequent culture of the cells
in vitro for six weeks resulted in the disappearance
of this band and a return to normal levels of
glucose-6-$PO_4$ dehydrogenase activity. This change,
combined with an increase in sex chromatin positive cells in the culture from 8 to 11 per cent to 25
to 35 per cent, the usual range in cells derived from
females after 16 weeks' gestation, suggests that X
chromosome inactivation might be taking place in

212

vitro similar to changes in vivo.[232]

Studies of arylsulfatase A activity for metachromatic leukodystrophy in cultured amniotic-fluid cells demonstrate developmental enzyme change with increasing length of gestation. Kaback et al.[70] have shown that arylsulfatase A activity appears to rise significantly from low activity in cultured fetal fibroblasts, to increased activity in cultured amniotic-fluid cells of the fetus, and to the most marked activity in maternal cultured skin fibroblasts. A similar sequence of increasing activity related to gestational age has been noted for $\beta$-galactosidase.[70] In contrast cultured amniotic-fluid cells and maternal cultured skin fibroblasts had equal $\beta$-D-N-acetylglucosaminidase activity, but significantly more activity than cultured fetal fibroblasts.

Nadler[232] has also shown that no appreciable differences in the activity of a number of enzymes (alkaline and acid phosphatase, galactose-1-P-uridyltransferase, alpha-glucosidase, 6-phosphogluconic dehydrogenase, lactic dehydrogenase, $\beta$-glucuronidase and $\beta$-galactosidase) could be demonstrated with the use of cells obtained at various stages of pregnancy and from newborn infants and adults.

Normal standards and variations for enzyme activities gained from studies of cultured skin fibroblasts cannot necessarily be extrapolated back to amniotic-fluid cells. For example, cystathionine synthase activity has been found to be several times higher in cultured amniotic-fluid cells obtained between 12 and 20 weeks of gestation than in cultured skin fibroblasts.[92] On the other hand, we have found argininosuccinase activity in cultured amniotic-fluid cells to be only half as much as in cultured skin fibroblasts,[87] and ornithine-keto-acid transaminase activity also to be lower in cultured amniotic cells than in cultured skin fibroblasts.[103]

Many of the metabolic disorders discussed have either quantitative or qualitatitive changes of their lysosomes. The tissue-culture technic now provides a very useful way to study normal and abnormal lysosomal function. It appears, for example, that serial propagation of cells that become senescent in culture may be accompanied by a progressive increase in number and size of the lysosomes, and show profound degenerative changes.[245] It may prove wiser to express a single enzyme activity as a ratio with one or more of the other enzymes at a comparable time during gestation to determine more accurately relative rather than absolute deficiencies. O'Brien[11] has cautioned that using noncultured amniotic-fluid cells for enzyme (hexosaminidase) assay may be unreliable. Apparently, there may be very low activity of this enzyme in noncultured cells, whereas in cultured cells of the same line, appreciable activity may be found. This caution should help prevent the incorrect diagnosis of Tay–Sachs disease in utero. It is possible that an enzymatic defect differs qualitatively or quantitatively in several forms of a disorder. In Tay–Sachs disease, for example, hexosaminidase A activity is absent, but at least two other forms of Tay–Sachs disease have been described, one with both hexosaminidase components A and B absent, and the other having only partial deficiency of hexosaminidase A.[246] Since the several forms of Niemann–Pick disease appear to be due to different mutations, quantitative differences in sphingomyelinase-type activity would be expected. In fact evidence has recently been presented that there are at least two different sphingomyelinases in this disease.[247] In Gaucher's disease patients whose cells showed the least glucocerebrosidase activity had the most rapid progression of the disease,[175] whereas in those with relatively less severe glucocerebrosidase deficiency, hepatosplenomegaly developed *later* in life.

The relation between enzyme deficiency and the appearance of overt clinical disorder, although intriguing, serves to emphasize further the necessary cautions in the interpretation of prenatal diagnostic data. We have studied an infant whose sibling had metachromatic leukodystrophy and demonstrated the absence of arylsulfatase A activity in his urine at two days of age. A sural-nerve biopsy at three weeks of age showed the typical features of metachromatic leukodystrophy. His cultured skin fibroblasts at four months of age showed arylsulfatase A deficiency. This child appeared developmentally normal until 10 months of age, after which neurologic impairment became evident, and the clinical features of metachromatic leukodystrophy have subsequently appeared. As mentioned earlier, Kolodny et al. were able to make a diagnosis of Tay–Sachs disease at six weeks of age — several months before the clinical signs appeared.[60]

The extensive necessary consideration of some of the many other biochemical and cultural factors involved in prenatal genetic diagnoses can only briefly be alluded to in this paper. For example certain enzyme activities are subject to exogenous control, and therefore the constituents of the medium used in culture assumes an important role. Some end products of metabolism may repress the synthesis of certain enzymes,[241] although this control mechanism may operate infrequently in cultured mammalian cells. The presence of certain enzymes in the culture medium may prevent or complicate the detection of some accumulated product.

The continued cautious and informed interpretation of data provided for prenatal diagnosis is advocated, since it remains unclear to what degree the biochemical activities of cultured cells can safely be extrapolated to cells in vivo.

## ETHICS, ECONOMICS AND TRENDS

Prenatal diagnosis has raised new and important medical, ethical, moral, legal and theologic issues, at a time when there is increasing public concern for population growth, women's rights, the consequences of illegal abortions, the number of "unwanted" children and the discriminatory aspects of current abortion laws. With increasing acceptance of abortion, and limitation of family size, it is probable that some families will seek termination of pregnancies that involve less severely affected fetuses, or those with disorders that are treatable to some extent. At present some difference of opinion would be expected about the propriety of interruption of a pregnancy for galactosemia or pyridoxine-responsive homocystinuria, but in the future, less reluctance for intervention under these circumstances is likely. In particular this will be true when treatment cannot completely assure normality, or when treatment is prolonged, detailed or expensive. It is also likely that abortion may be chosen for disorders of uncertain severity. Most people would probably prefer abortion for a fetus with a chromosome constitution of XYY, despite the uncertainty concerning the pathologic significance of this karyotype. It can in fact be anticipated that families will not want to risk any departure from the normal karyotype in their offspring. Finally, the ability to diagnose carrier states in utero provides the means to eradicate certain hereditary diseases, an approach that society might consider more seriously within a decade or two.

A leading factor bearing on these decisions for abortion may continue to be the significant complication frequency of therapeutic abortions in the second trimester, through hysterotomy or the introduction of hypertonic saline.[248] Improvements in technic here, possibly the use of the prostaglandins,[249] are crucial since it seems unlikely that amniocentesis can be done much earlier without considerable risk. Ideally, the establishment of a national registry could serve to collect and disseminate information from all the prenatal diagnostic units in the country, with special emphasis on immediate and long-term maternal and fetal risks. Co-ordinated efforts could help to standardize biochemical and cultural methods to provide a basis for the comparative critical evaluation of the accumulating data. During the development of these regional and national co-operative programs it may prove best for selected laboratories to provide specific diagnostic assays to aid in the useful centralization of facilities.

The proper impartial role of the obstetrician or geneticist is to provide informed counsel to the family about the nature and prognosis of the disorder, and the risk that the fetus will be affected. The decision for amniocentesis and subsequent intervention for an affected fetus will be made primarily by the family (and certainly an occasional family may for particular circumstances not desire amniocentesis in a high-risk situation). It seems inevitable that an occasion will eventually arise where one of a twin pair is found before birth to have a chromosomal abnormality. Whether or not to abort both these infants will be the difficult decision faced by the family and their physician. The parents should also be made aware that congenital abnormalities and other disorders cannot at present be diagnosed in utero.

It behooves the physician to remain impartial in counseling. Although society may have to bear the financial burden for long-term institutional care of a retarded child, it seems essential that society also remain impartial at this early point in the development of prenatal diagnosis, although ultimately it is likely to be involved to some degree.

216

Regarding the chromosomal indications for amniocentesis, much depends on the true magnitude of the risk of the procedure. If further experience confirms the risk to be very low for mother or fetus, it may be appropriate to offer this test to pregnant women of the group from 35 to 39 years of age as well as those over 40. On the basis of mongolism alone, a strong economic argument can be made for such a course. The latest data for Massachusetts[250] (1954-65) are consistent with the national figures, and allow the estimate that among the 90,645 live births in Massachusetts in 1968, probably 28 infants with mongolism occurred among the 6885 born to women 35 to 39 years of age, and 26 among the 2025 births in women 40 or older. Almost all persons with mongolism are institutionalized sooner or later in Massachusetts. Experience in the Walter E. Fernald State School for retarded children has been that about 1/3 are institutionalized in infancy, 1/3 at around the age of 10, and 1/3 at around the age of 30. We can estimate conservatively that, on the average, the remaining years of care in an institution would cost about $60,000 at current prices. Since close to 3000 patients with mongolism are institutionalized in Massachusetts today, the computed cost for their expected lifetime care approximates $180,000,000. The care of the 54 infants with mongolism estimated for 1968 only from pregnancies in women 35 years of age or older will cost the state at least $3,240,000.

Finally, if the risk of amniocentesis is indeed as low as appears, and the overall frequency of a serious chromosome disorder is about 1:200 live births,[143] the possibility arises that all pregnant women should be offered this diagnostic test. An economic argument cannot be fashioned for this proposition since many of the chromosome disorders, such as Turner's and Klinefelter's syndromes, would not require institutional care, but no one would question their cost in the other terms. It might become possible to screen amniotic fluid or cells for many metabolic disorders, though these in the sum would still not approach the frequency of chromosome disorders. Additional diseases of connective tissue, amino acid metabolism, glycogen storage, new lipidoses and hemolytic anemias will doubtless be added to the list. It is to be hoped that it will become possible to distinguish affected from

217

unaffected males for more X-linked disorders. Certain signs of various other autosomal dominant traits may become recognizable in amniotic-fluid cells.

A new dimension has been added to the traditional role of the physician, who is now able to predict diseases accurately before birth and to provide the means of preventing the birth of a child with mental defect or fatal disease. Our present responsibility is to establish safe technics and reliable data, which can then provide the required sound basis for legal, governmental, theologic and other considerations. Certainly, the challenge of these new responsibilities should not be the sole province of physicians, but one that must be shared with society.

## CONCLUSIONS

The advent of prenatal diagnosis through amniocentesis represents the most important advance so far attained in the prevention of the births of infants with irreparable genetic mental defect and fatal genetic disease. Genetic counseling in an increasing number of diseases can now be based upon actual diagnoses in utero instead of calculated probability risks. Although transabdominal amniocentesis at 14 to 16 weeks' gestation has been done without any apparent untoward result to fetus or mother in over 300 cases, the most careful evaluation of short-term and long-term follow-up study is necessary before any unreserved endorsement of this technic.

The prenatal diagnosis of chromosomal disorders has become the most numerically important group. Screening by amniocentesis is clearly feasible and indicated for cytogenetic disorders at least in women above 40 years of age. It should be emphasized that for the vast majority of women, these prenatal studies will serve as reassurance that their offspring will be chromosomally normal. The rational management of sex-linked diseases depends upon specific diagnosis in utero, which is now possible in only three disorders. For the remainder any action taken will depend upon accurate determination of fetal sex. Specific intrauterine diagnoses among the sphingolipidoses, mucopolysaccharidoses, amino acid and other miscellaneous disorders can now be definitively made. In these groups of inborn errors of metabolism invariably a family history of the particular disease is the reason for diagnostic amniocentesis. These inborn errors of metabolism, however, are too rare for routine screening at present.

A clear understanding of the multiple biochemical and cultural considerations involved in prenatal diagnoses is considered crucial to the informed interpretation of the data. Careful separation of heterozygous from homozygous states requires special emphasis. Through regional and national co-operative programs it should be possible to standardize technics and to provide specialized facilities in selected laboratories.

The medical, moral, legal and economic issues, problems and implications that have been raised will require extensive study over time. To assure continued progress it will be necessary to make rigorous efforts to maintain the high-quality control of data accumulation, to seek methodologic and technologic refinements and to exercise constant surveillance of the outcome and risks to mother and baby. Moreover, the challenge of these new responsibilities must be shared with society.

We are indebted to Drs. Raymond A. Adams, Sydney S. Gellis and John W. Grover for helpful comments on this paper.

## REFERENCES

1. Barr ML, Bertram EG: A morphological distinction between neurones of the male and female, and the behaviour of the nucleolar satellite during accelerated nucleoprotein synthesis. Nature (London) 163:676-677, 1949
2. Fuchs F, Riis P: Antenatal sex determination. Nature (London) 177:330, 1956
3. Serr DM, Sachs L, Danon M: Diagnosis of sex before birth using cells from the amniotic fluid. Bull Res Council Israel 58:137-138, 1955
4. Shettles LB: Nuclear morphology of cells in human amniotic fluid in relation to sex of infant. Amer J Obstet Gynec 71:834-838, 1956
5. Makowski EL, Prem KA, Kaiser IH: Detection of sex of fetuses by the incidence of sex chromatin body in nuclei of cells in amniotic fluid. Science 123:542-543, 1956
6. James F: Sexing foetuses by examination of amniotic fluid. Lancet 1:202-203, 1956
7. Steele MW, Breg WR Jr: Chromosome analysis of human amniotic-fluid cells. Lancet 1:383-385, 1966
8. Jacobson CB, Barter RH: Intrauterine diagnosis and management of genetic defects. Amer J Obstet Gynec 99:796-807, 1967
9. Nadler HL: Antenatal detection of hereditary disorders. Pediatrics 42:912-918, 1968
10. Valenti C, Schutta EF, Kehaty T: Cytogenetic diagnosis of Down's syndrome in utero. JAMA 207:1513-1515, 1969
11. Proceedings of the Conference on Antenatal Diagnosis, University of Chicago, June 11-12, 1970 (in press)
12. Littlefield JW, Goldstein S, Shih V: Somatic cell culture and birth defects. Proceedings of Third International Conference on Congenital Malformations, The Hague, Netherlands, September 7-13, 1969 (in press)

219

13. Plentl AA: Formation and circulation of amniotic fluid. Clin Obstet Gynec 9:427-439, 1966
14. Fuchs F: Volume of amniotic fluid at various stages of pregnancy. Clin Obstet Gynec 9:449-460, 1966
15. Bonsnes RW: Composition of amniotic fluid. Clin Obstet Gynec 9:440-448, 1966
16. Ostergard DR: The physiology and clinical importance of amniotic fluid: a review. Obstet Gynec Survey 25:297-319, 1970
17. Van Leeuwen L, Jacoby H, Charles D: Exfoliative cytology of amniotic fluid. Acta Cytol 9:442-445, 1965
18. Dancis J: The antepartum diagnosis of genetic diseases. J Pediat 72:301-302, 1968
19. Nadler HL: Prenatal detection of genetic defects. J Pediat 74:132-143, 1969
20. Seppälä M, Ruoslahti E, Tallberg Th: Genetical evidence for, maternal origin of amniotic proteins. Ann Med Exp Biol Fenn 44:6-7, 1966
21. Dancis J, Lind J, Vara P: Transfer of proteins across the human placenta, The Placenta and Fetal Membranes. Edited by C A Villee. Baltimore, Williams and Wilkins Company, 1960, pp 185-187
22. Brzezinski A, Sadovsky E, Shafrir E: Electrophoretic distribution of proteins in amniotic fluid and in maternal and fetal serum. Amer J Obstet Gynec 82:800-803, 1961
23. *Idem:* Protein composition of early amniotic fluid and fetal serum with a case of bis-albuminemia. Amer J Obstet Gynec 89:488-494, 1964
24. Freda VJ: The Rh problem in obstetrics and a new concept of its management using amniocentesis and spectrophotometric scanning of amniotic fluid. Amer J Obstet Gynec 92:341-374, 1965
25. Queenan JT, Adams DW: Amniocentesis for prenatal diagnosis of erythroblastosis fetalis. Obstet Gynec 25:302-307, 1965
26. Queenan JT: Amniocentesis and transamniotic fetal transfusion for Rh disease. Clin Obstet Gynec 9:491-507, 1966
27. Creasman WT, Lawrence RA, Thiede HA: Fetal complications of amniocentesis. JAMA 204:949-952, 1968
28. Nadler HL, Gerbie AB: Role of amniocentesis in the intrauterine detection of genetic disorders. New Eng J Med 282:596-599, 1970
29. Riis P, Fuchs F: Antenatal determination of foetal sex in prevention of hereditary diseases. Lancet 2:180-182, 1960
30. Pauls F, Boutros P: The value of placental localization prior to amniocentesis. Obstet Gynec 35:175-177, 1970
31. Gottesfeld KR, Thompson HE, Holmes JH, et al: Ultrasonic placentography — a new method for placental localization. Amer J Obstet Gynec 96:538-547, 1970
32. Donald I: Sonar as a method of studying prenatal development. J Pediat 75:326-333, 1969
33. Campbell S: The prediction of fetal maturity by ultrasonic measurement of the biparietal diameter. J Obstet Gynaec Brit Comm 76:603-609, 1969
34. Hellman LM, Duffus GM, Donald I, et al: Safety of diagnostic ultrasound in obstetrics. Lancet 1:1133-1135, 1970
35. Smyth MG: Animal toxicity studies with ultrasounds at diagnostic power levels, Diagnostic Ultrasound: Proceedings of the First International Conference, University of Pittsburgh, 1965. Edited by CC Grossman. Philadelphia, JB Lippincott Company, 1966, pp 296-299
36. Liley AW: The technique and complications of amniocentesis. New Zeal Med J 59:581-586, 1960
37. Freda VJ: Recent obstetrical advances in the Rh problem: antepartum management, amniocentesis, and experience with hysterotomy and surgery in utero. Bull NY Acad Med 42:474-503, 1966

220

38. Burnett RG, Anderson WR: The hazards of amniocentesis. J Iowa M Soc 58:130-137, 1968
39. Wiltchik SG, Schwarz RH, Emich JP Jr: Amniography for placental localization. Obstet Gynec 28:641-645, 1966
40. Berner HW Jr: Amniography, an accurate way to localize the placenta: a comparison with soft-tissue placentography. Obstet Gynec 29:200-206, 1967
41. Fuchs F: Genetic information from amniotic fluid constituents. Clin Obstet Gynec 9:565-573, 1966
42. Valenti C, Kehaty T: Culture of cells obtained by amniocentesis. J Lab Clin Med 73:355-358, 1969
43. Alvarez H: Diagnosis of hydatidiform mole by transabdominal placental biopsy. Amer J Obstet Gynec 95:538-541, 1966
44. Sato H, Kadotani T: Fetal skin biopsy. JAMA 212:323, 1970
45. Littlefield JW: The pregnancy at risk for a genetic disorder. New Eng J Med 282:627-628, 1970
46. *Idem:* Prenatal diagnosis and therapeutic abortion. New Eng J Med 280:722-723, 1969
47. Brady RO, Gal AE, Bradley RM, et al: Enzymatic defect in Fabry's disease: ceramidetrihexosidase deficiency. New Eng J Med 276:1163-1167, 1967
48. Matalon R, Dorfman A, Dawson G, et al: Glycolipid and mucopolysaccharide abnormality in fibroblasts of Fabry's Disease. Science 164:1522-1523, 1969
49. Kint JA: Fabry's Disease: alpha-galactosidase deficiency. Science 167:1268-1269, 1970
50. The Metabolic Basis of Inherited Disease. Second edition. Edited by JB Stanbury, JB Wyngaarden, DS Fredrickson. New York, McGraw-Hill Book Company, 1966
51. Brady RO, Kanfer JN, Shapiro D: Metabolism of glucocerebro sides. II. Evidence of an enzymatic deficiency in Gaucher's disease. Biochem Biophys Res Commun 18:221-225, 1965
52. Brady RO, Kanfer JN, Bradley RM, et al: Demonstration of a deficiency of glucocerebroside-cleaving enzyme in Gaucher's disease. J Clin Invest 45:1112-1115, 1966
53. Suzuki K, Chen GC: Brain ceramide hexosides in Tay-Sachs disease and generalized gangliosidosis ($G_{M1}$-gangliosidosis). J Lipid Res 8:105-113, 1967
54. Suzuki Y, Jacob JC, Suzuki K: A case of $G_{M2}$-gangliosidosis with total hexosaminidase deficiency. Neurology 20:388, 1970
55. O'Brien J: Generalized gangliosidosis. J Pediat 75:167-186, 1969
56. Suzuki K, Suzuki K, Kamoshita S: Chemical pathology of $G_{M1}$ gangliosidosis (generalized gangliosidosis). J Neuropath Exp Neurol 28:25-73, 1969
57. Sloan HR, Uhlendorf BW, Jacobson CB, et al: $\beta$-galactosidase in tissue culture derived from human skin and bone marrow: enzyme defect in $G_{M1}$ gangliosidosis. Pediat Res 3:532-537, 1969
58. *Idem:* $\beta$-galactosidase deficiency in $G_{M1}$ gangliosidosis: enzymatic and histochemical studies in tissue culture. Pediat Res 3:368, 1969
59. Eeg-Olofsson O, Kristensson K, Sourander P, et al: Tay-Sachs disease: a generalized metabolic disorder. Acta Paediat Scand 55:546-562, 1966
60. Kolodny EG, Uhlendorf BS, Quirk JM, et al: Gangliosides in cultured skin fibroblasts: accumulation in Tay Sachs disease. Presented at the Twelfth International Congress on Biochemistry of Lipids, Athens, Greece, September 7-11, 1969, p 39
61. Okada S, O'Brien JS: Tay-Sachs disease: generalized absence of a beta D-N-acetylhexosaminidase component. Science 165:698-700, 1969
62. Sandhoff K: Variation of $\beta$-N-acetylhexosaminidase-pattern in Tay-Sachs disease. FEBS Letters 4:351-354, 1969
63. Shneck L, Friedland J, Valenti C, et al: Prenatal diagnosis of Tay-Sachs disease. Lancet 1:582-584, 1970
64. O'Brien JS, Okada S, Chen A, et al: Tay-Sachs disease: detec-

221

tion of heterozygotes and homozygotes by serum hexosaminidase assay. New Eng J Med 283:15-20, 1970

65. Sandhoff K, Andreae U, Jatzkewitz H: Deficient hexosaminidase activity in an exceptional case of Tay-Sachs disease with additional storage of kidney globoside in visceral organs. Life Sci 7: 283-288, 1968

66. Austin J, Armstrong D, Shearer L: Metachromatic form of diffuse cerebral sclerosis: V. The nature and significance of low sulfatase activity: a controlled study of brain, liver and kidney in four patients with metachromatic leukodystrophy (MLD). Arch Neurol (Chicago) 13:593-614, 1965

67. Jatzkewitz H, Mehal E: Cerebroside-sulphatase and arylsulphatase A deficiency in metachromatic leukodystrophy (ML). J Neurochem 16:19-28, 1969

68. Murphy JV, Wolfe HL, Moser HW: Multiple sulfatase deficiencies in a variant form of metachromatic leukodystrophy, Lipid Storage Disease: Enzymatic defects and clinical implications. Edited by J Bernsohn. New York, Academic Press (in press)

69. Porter MT, Fluharty AL, Kihara H: Metachromatic leukodystrophy: arylsulfatase-A deficiency in skin fibroblast cultures. Proc Nat Acad Sci USA 62:887-891, 1969

70. Kaback MM, Howell RR: Infantile metachromatic leukodystrophy: heterozygote detection in skin fibroblasts and possible applications to intrauterine diagnosis. New Eng J Med 282:1336-1340, 1970

71. Holtz AI, Uhlendorf BW, Fredrickson DS: Persistence of a lipid defect in tissue cultures derived from patients with Niemann-Pick disease. Fed Proc 23:128, 1964

72. Schneck L, Volk BW: Clinical manifestations of Tay-Sachs disease and Niemann-Pick disease, Inborn Disorders of Sphingolipid Metabolism: Proceedings of the Third International Symposium on the Cerebral Sphingolipidoses. Edited by SM Aronson, BW Volk. Oxford, Pergamon Press, 1967, pp 403-411

73. Sloan HR, Uhlendorf BW, Kanfer JN, et al: Deficiency of sphingomyelin-cleaving enzyme activity in tissue cultures derived from patients with Niemann-Pick disease. Biochem Biophys Res Commun 34:582-588, 1969

74. Uhlendorf BW, Holtz AI, Mock MB, et al: Persistence of a metabolic defect in tissue culture derived from patients with Niemann-Pick disease, Inborn Disorders of Sphingolipid Metabolism: Proceedings of the Third International Symposium on the Cerebral Sphingolipidoses. Edited by SM Aronson, BW Volk. Oxford, Pergamon Press, 1967, pp 403-411

75. Kahlke W: Heredopathia atactica polyneuritiformis (Refsum's disease), Lipids and Lipidoses. Edited by G Shettler. New York, Springer-Verlag, 1967, pp 352-381

76. Herndon JH Jr, Steinberg D, Uhlendorf BW, et al: Refsum's disease: characterization of the enzyme defect in cell culture. J Clin Invest 48:1017-1032, 1969

77. Herndon JH Jr, Steinberg D, Uhlendorf BW: Refsum's disease: defective oxidation of phytanic acid in tissue cultures derived from homozygotes and heterozygotes. New Eng J Med 281: 1034-1038, 1969

78. MacBrinn M, Okada S, Woollacott M, et al: Beta-galactosidase deficiency in the Hurler syndrome. New Eng J Med 281:338-343, 1969

79. Ho MW, O'Brien JS: Hurler's syndrome: deficiency of a specific beta galactosidase isoenzyme. Science 165:611-613, 1969

80. McKusick VA: Heritable Disorders of Connective Tissue. Third edition. St. Louis, CV Mosby Company, 1966, pp 325-399

81. Danes BS, Bearn AG: Hurler's syndrome: a genetic study in cell culture. J Exp Med 123:1-16, 1966

82. Matalon R, Dorfman A: Acid mucopolysaccharides in cultured human fibroblasts. Lancet 2:838-841, 1969

222

83. Fratantoni JC, Neufeld EF, Uhlendorf BW, et al: Intrauterine diagnosis of the Hurler and Hunter syndromes. New Eng J Med 280:686-688, 1969
84. Matalon R, Dorfman A, Nadler HL, et al: A chemical method for the antenatal diagnosis of mucopolysaccharidoses. Lancet 1: 83-84, 1970
85. Fratantoni JC, Hall CW, Neufeld EF: The defect in Hurler and Hunter syndromes. II. Deficiency of specific factors involved in mucopolysaccharide degradation. Proc Nat Acad Sci USA 64: 360-366, 1969
86. Shih VE, Littlefield JW, Moser HW: Argininosuccinase deficiency in fibroblasts cultured from patients with argininosuccinic aciduria. Biochem Genet 3:81-83, 1969
87. Shih VE, Littlefield JW: Argininosuccinase activity in amniotic-fluid cells. Lancet 2:45, 1970
88. Tedesco TA, Mellman WJ: Argininosuccinate synthetase activity and citrulline metabolism in cells cultured from a citrullinemic subject. Proc Nat Acad Sci USA 57:829-834, 1967
89. Schulman JD, Wong VG, Bradley KH, et al: Cystinosis: biochemical, morphological and clinical studies. Pediat Res 4:379, 1970
90. Schneider JA, Rosenbloom FM, Bradley KH, et al: Increased free-cystine content of fibroblasts cultured from patients with cystinosis. Biochem Biophys Res Commun 29:527-531, 1967
91. Hummeler K, Zajac BA, Genel M, et al: Human cystinosis: in tracellular deposition of cystine. Science 168:859-860, 1970
92. Uhlendorf BW, Mudd SH: Cystathionine synthase in tissue culture derived from human skin: enzyme defect in homocystinuria. Science 160:1007-1009, 1968
93. Nadler HL, Gerbie AB: Enzymes in noncultured amniotic fluid cells. Amer J Obstet Gynec 103:710-712, 1969
94. Dancis J, Hutzler J, Cox RP, et al: Familial hyperlysinemia with lysine-ketoglutarate reductase deficiency. J Clin Invest 48:1447-1452, 1969
95. Hsia YR, Scully KJ, Rosenberg LE: Inherited proprionyl-CoA carboxylase deficiency in "ketotic hyperglycinemia." Presented at the annual meeting of the American Pediatric Society and the Society for Pediatric Research, Atlantic City, April 29-May 2, 1970, p 26
96. Seegmiller JD, Westall RG: The enzyme defect in maple syrup urine disease (branched chain ketoaciduria). J Ment Defic Res 11:288-294, 1967
97. Dancis J, Jansen V, Hutzler J, et al: The metabolism of leucine in tissue culture of skin fibroblasts of maple-syrup-urine disease. Biochim Biophys Acta 77:523-524, 1963
98. Snyderman SE: Maple syrup urine disease, Amino Acid Metabolism and Genetic Variation. Edited by WL Nyhan. New York, McGraw-Hill Book Company, 1967, pp 171-183
99. Dancis J, Hutzler J, Cox RP: Enzyme defect in skin fibroblasts in intermittent branched-chain ketonuria and in maple syrup urine disease. Biochem Med 2:407-411, 1969
100. Morrow G III, Mellman WJ, Barness LA, et al: Propionate metabolism in cells cultured from a patient with methylmalonic acidemia. Pediat Res 3:217-219, 1969
101. Rosenberg LE, Lilljeqvist A-C, Hsia YE, et al: Vitamin B$_{12}$ dependent methylmalonicaciduria: defective B$_{12}$ metabolism in cultured fibroblasts. Biochem Biophys Res Comm 37:607-614, 1969
102. Morrow G III, Schwarz RH, Hallock JA: Prenatal detection of methylmalonic acidemia. J Pediat 77:120-123, 1970
103. Shih VE, Schulman JD: Ornithine-ketoacid transaminase activity in human skin and amniotic fluid cell culture. Clin Chim Acta 27:73-75, 1970
104. Durand P, Borrone C, Della Cella G: Fucosidosis. J Pediat 75: 665-674, 1969

105. Van Hoof F, Hers HG: Mucopolysaccharidosis by absence of α-fucosidase. Lancet 1:1198, 1968
106. Leroy J, Ho MW, O'Brien JS: Personal communication
107. Nitowsky HM, Grunefeld A: Lysosomal α-glucosidase in type II glycogenosis: activity in leukocytes and cell cultures in relation to genotype. J Lab Clin Med 69:472-484, 1967
108. Dancis J, Hutzler J, Lynfield J, et al: Absence of acid maltase in glycogenesis type 2 (Pompe's disease) in tissue culture. Amer J Dis Child 117:108-111, 1969
109. Nadler HL, Messina AM: In-utero detection of type-II glycogenosis (Pompe's disease). Lancet 2:1277-1278, 1969
110. Cox RP, Douglas G, Hutzler J, et al: In-utero detection of Pompe's disease. Lancet 1:893, 1970
111. Howell RR, Kaback MM, Brown BI: Type IV glycogen storage disease: branching enzyme deficiency in skin fibroblasts and possible heterozygote detection. Presented at the annual meeting of the American Pediatric Society and the Society for Pediatric Research, Atlantic City, April 29-May 2, 1970, p 130
112. Krooth RS, Weinberg AN: Studies on cell lines developed from the tissues of patients with galactosemia. J Exp Med 113:1155-1172, 1961
113. Nadler HL: Antenatal detection of hereditary disorders. Pediatrics 42:912-918, 1968
114. Russell JD: Variation of UDP Glu: α-DGal-1-P-uridyl transferase activity during growth of cultured fibroblasts, Galactosemia. Edited by DY-Y Hsia. Springfield, Illinois, Charles C Thomas, 1969, pp 204-212
115. Öckerman P-A: Mannosidosis: isolation of oligosaccharide storage material from brain. J Pediat 75:360-365, 1969
116. Kjellman B, Gamstorp I, Brun A, et al: Mannosidosis: a clinical and histopathologic study. J Pediat 75:366-373, 1969
117. Blass JP, Schulman JD, Uhlendorf BW, et al: Inherited abnormalities in pyruvic acid metabolism in fibroblasts from patients with neurologic diseases. Presented at the First Annual Meeting of the American Neurochemical Society, Albuquerque, New Mexico, March 16-18, 1970, p 30
118. Blass JP, Avigan J, Uhlendorf BW: A defect in pyruvate decarboxylase in a child with an intermittent movement disorder. J Clin Invest 49:423-432, 1970
119. Davidson RG, Nitowsky HM, Childs B: Demonstration of two populations of cells in the human female heterozygous for glucose-6-phosphate dehydrogenase variants. Proc Nat Acad Sci USA 50:481-485, 1963
120. Krooth RS, Howell RR, Hamilton HB: Properties of acatalasic cells growing in vitro. J Exp Med 115:313-328, 1962
121. Jeffcoate TNA, Fliegner JRH, Russell SH, et al: Diagnosis of the adrenogenital syndrome before birth. Lancet 2:553-555, 1965
122. Cathro DM, Bertrand J, Coyle MG: Antenatal diagnosis of adrenocortical hyperplasia. Lancet 1:732, 1969
123. Nichols J: Antenatal diagnosis of adrenocortical hyperplasia. Lancet 1:1151-1152, 1969
124. Nichols J, Gibson GG: Antenatal diagnosis of the adrenogenital syndrome. Lancet 2:1068-1069, 1969
125. Merkatz IR, New MI, Peterson RE, et al: Prenatal diagnosis of adrenogenital syndrome by amniocentesis. J Pediat 75:977-982, 1969
126. Danes BS, Bearn AG: Cell culture and the Chediak-Higashi syndrome. Lancet 2:65-67, 1967
127. Romeo G, Kaback MM, Glenn BL, et al: The enzymatic defect in congenital erythropoietic porphyria: demonstration in heterozygotes and in nonerythropoietic tissue of homozygotes. Presented at the annual meeting of the American Pediatric Society and the Society for Pediatric Research, Atlantic City, April 29-May 2, 1970, p 76
128. Danes BS, Bearn AG: A genetic cell marker in cystic fibrosis of

224

the pancreas. Lancet 1:1061-1063, 1968

129. *Idem:* Cystic fibrosis of the pancreas: a study in cell culture. J Exp Med 129:775-793, 1969

130. Nadler HL, Swae MA, Wodnicki JM, et al: Cultivated amniotic-fluid cells and fibroblasts derived from families with cystic fibrosis. Lancet 2:84-85, 1969

131. Gibbs GE, Griffin GD: Beta glucuronidase activity in skin components of children with cystic fibrosis. Science 167:993-994, 1970

132. Matalon R, Dorfman A: Acid mucopolysaccharides in cultured fibroblasts of cystic fibrosis of the pancreas. Biochem Biophys Res Commun 33:954-958, 1968

133. Leroy JG, DeMars RI, Opitz JM: "I-cell" disease, The First Conference on the Clinical Delineation of Birth Defects. Part 4. Skeletal Dysplasias (Birth Defects Original Article Series Vol 5, No. 4). Edited by D Bergsma. New York, The National Foundation, 1969, pp 174-189

134. Leroy JG, DeMars RI: Mutant enzymatic and cytological phenotypes in cultured human fibroplasts. Science 157:804-806, 1967

135. DeMars R, Leroy JG: The remarkable cells cultured from a human with Hurler's syndrome, In Vitro. Vol 2. Phenotypic Expression. Edited by CJ Dawe. Baltimore, Williams and Wilkins, 1966, pp 107-118

136. Dancis J, Cox RP, Berman PH, et al: Cell population density and phenotypic expression of tissue culture fibroblasts from heterozygotes of Lesch-Nyhan's disease (inosinate pyrophosphorylase deficiency). Biochem Genet 3:609-615, 1969

137. Berman PH, Balis ME, Dancis J: A method for the prenatal diagnosis of congenital hyperuricemia. J Pediat 75:488-491, 1969

138. Nadler HL, Egan TJ: Deficiency of lysosomal acid phosphatase: a new familial metabolic disorder. New Eng J Med 282:302-307, 1970

139. Matalon R, Dorfman A: The accumulation of hyaluronic acid in cultured fibroblasts of the Marfan syndrome. Biochem Biophys Res Commun 32:150-154, 1968

140. Krooth RS: Properties of diploid cell strains developed from patients with an inherited abnormality of uridine biosynthesis. Sympos Quant Biol 29:189-212, 1964

141. Cleaver JE: Defective repair replication of DNA in xeroderma pigmentosum. Nature (London) 218:652-656, 1968

142. *Idem:* Personal communication

143. Court Brown WM: Males with an XYY sex chromosome complement. J Med Genet 5:341-359, 1968

144. Taylor AI: Autosomal trisomy syndromes: a detailed study of 27 cases of Edwards' syndrome and 27 cases of Patau's syndrome. J Med Genet 5:227-252, 1968

145. Court Brown WM, Law P, Smith PG: Sex chromosome aneuploidy and parental age. Ann Hum Genet 33:1-11, 1969

146. Turpin R, Lejeune J: Human Afflictions and Chromosomal Aberrations. London, Pergamon Press, 1969

147. Collmann RD, Stoller A: A survey of mongoloid births in Victoria, Australia, 1942-57. Amer J Public Health 52:813-829, 1962

148. Carter CO, MacCarthy D: Incidence of mongolism and its diagnosis in the newborn, Brit J Soc Med 5:83-90, 1951

149. Penrose LS, Smith GF: Down's Anomaly. London, I and A Churchill, 1966

150. Turpin R, Lejeune J: Les Chromosomes Humaines: Caryotype normal et variations pathologiques. Paris, Gauthier Villar, 1965

151. Chromosomes in Medicine. Edited by JL Hamerton. London, Medical Advisory Committee, National Spastics Society, 1962 (Little Club Clinics in Developmental Medicine No 5), pp 137-180

152. Hamerton JI.: Chromosome segregation in three human interchanges, Chromosomes Today. Vol 1. Edited by CD Darlington, KR Lewis. Edinburgh, Oliver and Boyd, 1966, pp 237-252

225

153. *Idem:* Fetal sex. Lancet 1:516-517, 1970
154. *Idem:* Robertsonian translocations in man: evidence for prezygotic selection. Cytogenetics 7:260-276, 1968
155. Ford CE, Clegg HM: Reciprocal translocations. Brit Med Bull , 25:110-114, 1969
156. Hamerton JL: Reciprocal translocation in man, Chromosomes Today. Vol 2. Edited by CD Darlington, KR Lewis. Edinburgh, Oliver and Boyd, 1969, pp 21-32
157. Thiede HA, Creasman WT, Metcalfe S: Antenatal analysis of the human chromosomes. Amer J Obstet Gynec 94:589-590, 1966
158. Nelson MM, Emery AEH: Amniotic fluid cells: prenatal sex prediction and culture. Brit Med J 1:523-526, 1970
159. Bergadá C, Farias NE, Romero De Bahar BM, et al: Abnormal sex chromatin pattern in cryptorchidism, girls with short stature and other endocrine patients. Helv Paediat Acta 24:372-377, 1969
160. Klinger HP, Schwarzacher HG: The sex chromatin and heterochromatic bodies in human diploid and polyploid nuclei. J Biophys Biochem Cytol 8:345-364, 1960
161. Böök JA, Kjessler B, Santesson B: Karyotypes of cultured cells from foetal membranes of normal newborns. J Med Genet 5:224-226, 1968
162. Schlegel RJ, Neu RL, Leão JC, et al: Observations on the chromosomal cytological and anatomical characteristics of 75 human conceptuses. Cytogenetics 5:430-446, 1966
163. Fraccaro M, Gemzell CA, Lindsten J: Plasma level of growth hormone and chromosome complement in four patients with gonadal dysgenesis (Turner's syndrome). Acta Endocr (Kobenhavn) 34:496-507, 1960
164. Kohn G, Mayall BH, Miller ME, et al: Tetraploid-diploid mosaicism in a surviving infant. Pediat Res 1:461-469, 1967
165. Carr DH: Chromosome studies in abortuses and stillborn infants. Lancet 2:603-606, 1963
166. Waxman SH, Arakaki DT, Smith JB: Cytogenetics of fetal abortions. Pediatrics 39:425-432, 1967
167. Hughes EC, Csermely VT: Chromosome constitution of human endometrium. Amer J Obstet Gynec 93:777-792, 1965
168. Court Brown WM, Harnden DC, Jacobs PA, et al: Abnormalities of the sex chromosome complement in man. Med Res Counc Spec Res Series (London) 305:1-239, 1964
169. Carter CO, Evans KA: Risks of parents who have had one child with Down's syndrome (mongolism) having another child similarly affected. Lancet 2:785-788, 1961
170. Hamerton JL, Briggs SM, Giannelli F: Chromosome studies in detection of parents with high risk of second child with Down's Syndrome. Lancet 2:788-791, 1961
171. Seegmiller JE, Rosenbloom FM, Kelley WN: Enzyme defect associated with a sex-linked human neurological disorder and excessive purine synthesis. Science 155:1682-1684, 1967
172. DeMars R, Santo G, Felix JS: Lesch-Nyhan mutation: prenatal detection with amniotic fluid cells. Science 164:1303-1305, 1969
173. Fujimoto WY, Seegmiller JE, Uhlendorf BW, et al: Biochemical diagnosis of an X-linked disease in utero. Lancet 2:511-512, 1968
174. Zacharski LR, Bowie EJW, Titus JL: Cell-culture synthesis of a factor VIII-like activity. Mayo Clin Proc 44:784-792, 1969
175. Brady RO: Genetics and the sphingolipidoses. Med Clin N Amer 53:827-838, 1969
176. Crocker AC: The cerebral defect in Tay-Sachs disease and Niemann-Pick disease. J Neurochem 7:69-80, 1961
177. Austin J, Balasubramanian AS, Pattabiraman TN, et al: A controlled study of enzymic activities on three human disorders of glycolipid metabolism. J Neurochem 10:805-816, 1963
178. Mehl E, Jatzkewitz H: Evidence for a genetic block in metachromatic leukodystrophy. Biochem Biophy Commun 19:407-411, 1965

179. Austin J, Armstrong D, Shearer L, et al: Metachromatic form of diffuse cerebral sclerosis. VI. A rapid test for sulfatase A deficiency in metachromatic leukodystrophy urine. Arch Neurol (Chicago) 14:259-269, 1966
180. Percy AK, Brady RO: Metachromatic leukodystrophy: diagnosis with samples of venous blood. Science 161:594-595, 1968
181. Krabbe K: A new familial infantile form of diffuse brain-sclerosis. Brain 39:74-114, 1916
182. Mapes CA, Anderson RL, Sweeley CC: Galactosylgalactosylglucosylceramide: galactosyl hydrolase in normal human plasma and its absence in patients with Fabry's disease. FEBS Letters 7:180-181, 1970
183. Austin J: Studies in globoid (Krabbe) leukodystrophy. I. The significance of lipid abnormalities in white matter in 8 globoid and 13 control patients. Arch Neurol (Chicago) 9:207-231, 1963
184. Bachhawat BK, Austin J, Armstrong D: A cerebroside sulfotransferase deficiency in a human disorder of myelin. Biochem J 104:15c-17c, 1967
185. Eto Y, Suzuki K: Brain sphingoglycolipids in globoid-cell leukodystrophy. Presented at a meeting of the American Society for Neurochemistry, Albuquerque, New Mexico, March 16-18, 1970, p 42
186. Malone M: Deficiency in a degradative enzyme system in globoid leukodystrophy. Presented at a meeting of the American Society for Neurochemistry, Albuquerque, New Mexico, March 16-18, 1970, p 42
187. Myrianthopoulos NC, Aronson SM: Population dynamics of Tay-Sachs disease. I. Reproductive fitness and selection. Amer J Hum Genet 18:313-327, 1966
188. Shaw RF, Smith AP: Is Tay-Sachs disease increasing? Nature (London) 224:1213-1215, 1969
189. Kolodny EH, Brady RO, Volk BW: Demonstration of an alteration of ganglioside metabolism in Tay-Sachs disease. Biochem Biophys Res Commun 37:526-531, 1969
190. Wolfe LS, Callahan J, Fawcett JS, et al: $G_{M1}$-gangliosidosis without chondrodystrophy or visceromegaly. Neurology (Minneap) 20:23-44, 1970
191. Sacrez R, Juif JG, Gigonnet JM, et al: La maladie de Landing: ou idiotie amaurotique infantile précoce avec gangliosidose généralisée de type GM 1. Pediatrie 22:143-162, 1967
192. Okada S, O'Brien JS: Generalized gangliosidosis: beta-galactosidase deficiency. Science 160:1002-1004, 1968
193. Kint JA, Dacremont G, Vlietinck R: Type-II $G_{M1}$ gangliosidosis? Lancet 2:108-109, 1969
194. Thomas GH: Beta-D-galactosidase in human urine: deficiency in generalized gangliosidosis. J Lab Clin Med 74:725-731, 1969
195. Schneck L, Volk BW, Saifer A: The gangliosidoses. Amer J Med 46:245-263, 1969
196. Symposium on the mucopolysaccharidoses. Amer J Med 47:661-747, 1969
197. Vaubel E: The form and function of synovial cells in tissue cultures. I. Morphology of cells under varying conditions. II. The production of mucin. J Exp Med 58:63-83, 85-95, 1933
198. Grossfeld H, Meyer K, Godman G: Differentiation of fibroblasts in tissue culture, as determined by mucopolysaccharide production. Proc Soc Exp Biol Med 88:31-35, 1955
199. Gains LM Jr: Synthesis of acid mucopolysaccharides and collagen in tissue cultures of fibroblasts. Bull Johns Hopkins Hosp 106:195-204, 1960
200. Danes BS, Bearn AG: Hurler's syndrome: demonstration of an inherited disorder of connective tissue in cell culture. Science 149:987-989, 1965
201. Milunsky A, Littlefield JW: Diagnostic limitations of metachromasia. New Eng J Med 281:1128-1129, 1969

227

202. Schafer IA, Silverman L, Sullivan JC, et al: Ascorbic acid deficiency in cultured human fibroblasts. J Cell Biol 34:83-95, 1967

203. Matalon R, Dorfman A: Hurler's syndrome: biosynthesis of acid mucopolysaccharides in tissue culture. Proc Nat Acad Sci USA 56:1310-1316, 1966

204. Antonopoulos CA, Gardell S, Szirmai JA, et al: Determination of glycosaminoglycans (mucopolysaccharides) from tissues on the microgram scale. Biochim Biophy Acta 83:1-19, 1964

205. Švejcar J, Robertson WVanB: Micro separation and determination of mammalian acidic glycosaminoglycans (mucopolysaccharides). Anal Biochem 18:333-350, 1967

206. Van Hoot F, Hers HG: The abnormalities of lysosomal enzymes in mucopolysaccharidoses. Europ J Biochem 7:34-44, 1968

207. Fratantoni JC, Hall CW, Neufeld EF: The defect in Hurler's and Hunter's syndromes: faulty degradation of mucopolysaccharide. Proc Nat Acad Sci USA 60:699-706, 1968

208. Idem: Hurler and Hunter syndromes: mutual correction of the defect in cultured fibroblasts. Science 162:570-572, 1968

209. Schafer IA, Sullivan JC, Švejcar J, et al: Study of the Hurler syndrome using cell culture: definition of the biochemical phenotype and the effect of ascorbic acid on the mutant cell. J Clin Invest 47:321-328, 1968

210. Idem: Vitamin C-induced increase of dermatan sulfate in cultured Hurler's fibroblasts. Science 153:1008-1010, 1966

211. Danes BS, Bearn AG: Hurler's syndrome: effect of retinol (Vitamin A alcohol) on cellular mucopolysaccharides in cultured human skin fibroblasts. J Exp Med 124:1181-1198, 1966

212. Danes BS, Queenan JT, Gadow EC, et al: Antenatal diagnosis of mucopolysaccharidoses. Lancet 1:946-947, 1970

213. Dingle JT, Webb M: Mucopolysaccharide metabolism in tissue culture. Cells and Tissues in Culture: Methods, biology and physiology. Vol 1. Edited by EN Willmer. New York, Academic Press, 1965, pp 353-396

214. Grossfeld H, Meyer K, Godman GC, et al: Mucopolysaccharides produced in tissue culture. J Biophys Biochem Cytol 3:391-396, 1957

215. Daniel MR, Dingle JT, Lucy JA: Cobalt-tolerance and mucopolysaccharide production in rat dermal fibroblasts in culture. Exp Cell Res 24:88-105, 1961

216. Levy HL, Shih VE, MacCready RA: Massachusetts Metabolic Disorders Screening Program, Proceedings of the Fogarty International Conference on Ethical Problems in Human Genetics, National Institutes of Health, Washington, D.C., May 18-19, 1970 (in press)

217. Gartler SM: Metabolic errors of the whole organism reflected in cell culture systems, Retention of Function Differentiation in Cultured Cells. Philadelphia, Wistar Institute Press, 1964 (Wistar Institute Symposium Monograph No 1), pp 63-69

218. Levy HL, Easterday CL, Montag PP, et al: Amino acids in amniotic fluid, Proceedings of the Conference on Antenatal Diagnosis, University of Chicago, June 11-12, 1970 (in press)

219. Levy HL, Montag PP: Free amino acids in human amniotic fluid: a quantitative study of ion-exchange chromatography. Pediat Res 3:113-120, 1969

220. Emery AEH, Burt D, Nelson MM, et al: Antenatal diagnosis and aminoacid composition of amniotic fluid. Lancet 1:1307-1308, 1970

221. Alpers JB, Wu R, Racker E: Regulatory mechanisms in carbohydrate metabolism. VI. Glycogen metabolism in HeLa cells. J Biol Chem 238:2274-2280, 1963

222. Cassady G, Cailliteau J: The amniotic fluid in anencephaly: preliminary report. Amer J Obstet Gynec 97:395-399, 1967

223. Liley AW: Errors in the assessment of hemolytic disease from amniotic fluid. Amer J Obstet Gynec 86:485-494, 1963
224. Willoughby HW, Henry JS Jr, Arronet GH: Amniotic fluid in a case of multiple congenital anomalies. Canad Med Ass J 101: 354-355, 1969
225. Nelson GM: Amniotic fluid phospholipid patterns in normal and abnormal pregnancies. Amer J Obstet Gynec 105:1072-1077, 1969
226. Berlin CM, Jacobson CB: Congenital anomalies associated with parental LSD ingestion. Pediat Res 4:377, 1970
227. Queenan JT, Gadow EC: Amniography for detection of congenital malformations. Obstet Gynec 35:648-657, 1970
228. Taysi K, Kistenmacher ML, Punnett HH, et al: Limitations of metachromasia as a diagnostic aid in pediatrics. New Eng J Med 281:1108-1111, 1969
229. Bartman J, Wiesmann U, Blanc WA: Ultrastructure of cultivated fibroblasts in cystic fibrosis of the pancreas. J Pediat 76:430-437, 1970
230. Danes BS, Bearn AG: Cystic fibrosis: distribution of mucopolysaccharides in fibroblast cultures. Biochem Biophys Res Commun 36:919-924, 1969
231. Pallavicini JC, Wiesmann U, Uhlendorf BW: Glycogen content of tissue culture fibroblasts from patients with cystic fibrosis and other heritable disorders. J Pediat 77:280-284, 1970
232. Nadler HL: Patterns of enzyme development utilizing cultivated human fetal cells derived from amniotic fluid. Biochem Genet 2: 119-126, 1968
233. Swift MR, Finegold MJ: Myotonic muscular dystrophy: abnormalities in fibroblast culture. Science 165:294-296, 1969
234. Krooth RS: Genetics of cultured somatic cells. Med Clin N Amer 53:795-811, 1969
235. Krooth RS, Darlington GA, Velazquez AA: The genetics of cultured mammalian cells. Ann Rev Genet 2:141-164, 1968
236. Kelley WN, Greene ML, Rosenbloom FM, et al: Hypoxanthineguanine, phosphoribosyltransferase deficiency in gout. Ann Intern Med 70:155-206, 1969
237. Goldstein S, Littlefield JW: Effect of insulin on the conversion of glucose-C-14-to C-14 $O_2$ by normal and diabetic fibroblasts in culture. Diabetes 18:545-549, 1969
238. Goldstein S: Lifespan of cultured cells in progeria. Lancet 1:424, 1969
239. Eagle H: Amino acid metabolism in mammalian cell cultures. Science 130:432-437, 1959
240. Levintow L, Eagle H: Biochemistry of cultured mammalian cells. Ann Rev Biochem 30:605-640, 1961
241. Eagle H: Metabolic controls in cultured mammalian cells. Science 148:42-51, 1965
242. Eagle H, Piez KA: Amino acids, protein synthesis and protein turnover in human cell cultures, Amino Acid Pools: Distribution, formation and function of free amino acids. Edited by JT Holden. Amsterdam, Elsevier Publishing Company, 1962, pp 694-705
243. DeMars R: Some studies of enzymes in cultivated human cells Nat Cancer Inst Monogr 13:181-193, 1964
244. De Luca C, Nitowsky HM: Variations in enzyme activities during the growth of mammalian cells in vitro: lactate and glucose-6-phosphate dehydrogenases. Biochim Biophys Acta 89:208-216, 1964
245. Robbins E, Levine EM, Eagle H: Morphologic changes accompanying senescence of cultured human diploid cells. J Exp Med 131:1211-1222, 1970
246. O'Brien JS: Five gangliosidoses. Lancet 2:805, 1969
247. Lowden JA, LaRamee MA: Sphingomyelinases in Niemann-Pick

disease. Presented at a meeting of the American Society for Neu-, rochemistry, Albuquerque, New Mexico, March 16-18, 1970, p 55

248. Schiffer MA: Induction of labor by intra-amniotic instillation of hypertonic solution for therapeutic abortion or intrauterine death. Obstet Gynec 33:729-736, 1969

249. Karim SMM, Filshie GM: Therapeutic abortion using prostaglandin F $\alpha$. Lancet 1:157-159, 1970

250. Fabia J: Illegitimacy and Down's syndrome. Nature (London) 221:1157-1158, 1969

# ANTENATAL DETECTION OF HEREDITARY DISORDERS

**Henry L. Nadler, M.D.**

ABSTRACT. Amniotic fluid cells obtained by trans-abdominal amniocentesis at various stages of pregnancy were successfully cultivated. The intra-uterine detection of Down's syndrome, galactosemia, and mucopolysaccharidosis was established utilizing the cultivated amniotic fluid cells. The use of this procedure increases the precision of genetic counseling and should stimulate the development of new approaches for the intra-uterine management of genetic defects. However, until considerably more experience is gained with these techniques, these procedures should be considered experimental in nature. *Pediatrics*, 42:912, 1968, Down's SYNDROME, GALACTOSEMIA, MUCOPOLYSACCHARIDOSIS, GENETIC DISORDERS, AMNIOCENTESIS, HEREDITARY DISORDERS.

THE successful utilization of the procedure of amniocentesis in the management of erythroblastosis fetalis has demonstrated both the feasibility and the potential usefulness of this procedure for the intra-uterine diagnosis and management of this genetic disorder.[1-3] Previous attempts to utilize amniotic fluid for the prenatal diagnosis of genetic disorders used desquamated fetal cells for sex chromatin analysis[4-7] in the antenatal determination of fetal sex. Riis and Fuchs[8] and Serr and Margolis[9] utilized sex chromatin analysis to manage pregnancies for two x-linked recessive disorders—hemophilia and muscular dystrophy. Jeffcoate, et al.[10] and Fuchs[11] have been able to establish the in utero diagnosis of the adrenogenital syndrome by

This study is supported by U.S. Public Health Grants 5 RO1 HD 02752 and TI AM 5186.

measuring the 17-ketosteroids and pregnanetriol level in amniotic fluid. Recently, Steele and Breg[12] and Jacobson and Barter[13] have demonstrated the ability to cultivate these desquamated cells in culture and to use them for the analysis of chromosomes.

The purpose of this study was to demonstrate the ability to cultivate fetal cells obtained by amniocentesis at various stages of pregnancy and to point out the potential usefulness of these cells for the intra-uterine detection of cytogenetic and biochemical disorders.

## METHODS

Abdominal amniocenteses were performed on 37 women at various stages during pregnancy. In the majority of patients (23), the indication for amniocentesis was the management of Rh incompatibility. In addition, amniotic fluid was obtained at the time of a cesarean section in three cases, prior to scheduled therapeutic abortions in seven cases, and for management of high risk pregnancies in two cases. Usually 5 to 10 cc of fluid was collected using a transabdominal approach. The fluid was centrifuged at 600 xg for 12 minutes, and the cell pellet was resuspended in one-half cubic centimeter of fetal calf serum. One-fourth cubic centimeter of cell suspension was placed in two 30 mm Falcon petri dishes and a cover slip was placed over the cells to immobilize them. After 20 to 30 minutes, 2 cc of Nutrient Mixture F10 containing 30% fetal calf serum* was added to each dish. The cells were placed in a 5% $CO_2$ atmosphere at 37°C and fed daily. After approximately 18 to 25 days, the cells were trypsinized and subcultured using a 04% trypsin-viokase solution. The cells were subcultured a second time after 3 to 5 days and could then be used for cytogenetic[14] and for biochemical analysis.[15–17]

## RESULTS

In Table I are summarized the results of 37 amniocenteses performed at specific times during pregnancy in 35 patients. Successful cultivation is defined as the ability to maintain the culture after two subcultures. Cells were successfully cultivated in 27 cases. In two cases, cultures could be maintained through only a single subculture, while in three cases, despite adequate growth of the primary culture, a successful subculture was not obtained. In five cases, no cell growth could be demonstrated. In four cases not successfully cultivated after 24 weeks of pregnancy, the amniotic fluid contained large amounts of red cells and high levels of bilirubin. Two of these amniocenteses were performed on the same woman, the second following an intra-uterine transfusion. In the one case not successfully cultivated at 10 weeks, the amniotic fluid was stored for 20 days prior to attempted cultivation. The duration of pregnancy was estimated from the history and physical examination performed by the obstetrician. The sex of the fetuses listed in Table I was determined by chromosome analysis of the cultivated amniotic fluid cells. In all cases the predicted sex was confirmed after delivery by examination of the external genitalia, and after therapeutic abortion by chromosome analysis of the cultured abortion material.

The clinical usefulness of this procedure is demonstrated by the following five cases.

### Case I

Mrs. R. K, a 25-year-old Caucasian female who is a known carrier of a D/G translocation (Fig. 1), was scheduled to have her pregnancy interrupted at 10 weeks for psychiatric indications. Immedi-

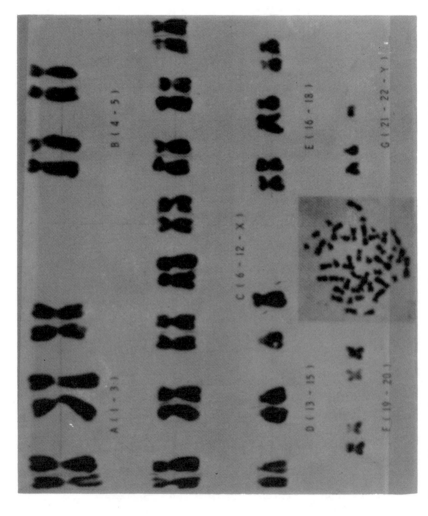

FIG. 1. Karyotype of Mrs. R. K., a D/G translocation carrier, derived from a peripheral blood culture.

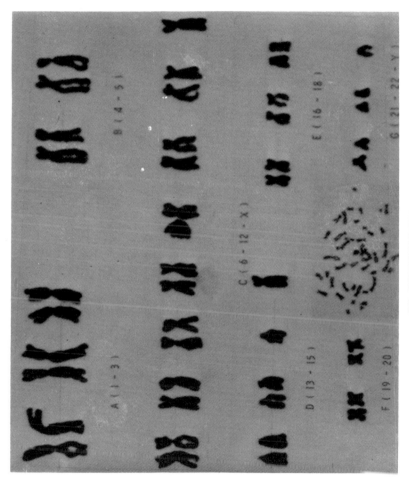

Fig. 2. Karyotype of fetus in Case I, derived from cultivated amniotic fluid cells demonstrating 46 chromosomes, XY, including D/G translocation (Down's syndrome).

235

ately prior to the therapeutic abortion (dilatation and curettage), 10 cc of amniotic fluid was obtained. Chromosome analysis of both the cultivated amniotic fluid cells and the material obtained at the time of the therapeutic abortion demonstrated the presence of 46 chromosomes, XY, including the D/G translocation (Fig. 2). This finding is consistent with the diagnosis of Down's syndrome.

## Case II

Mrs. S. T., a 28-year-old Caucasian female, was referred to an obstetrician for interruption of pregnancy by her family physician because of her history of having had a child with Down's syndrome. Chromosome analysis performed on the mother utilizing peripheral blood demonstrated the presence of 45 chromosomes, XX, including a D/G translocation. An amniocentesis was performed at 10 weeks of pregnancy. Chromosome analysis using cultivated amniotic fluid cells demonstrated the presence of 46 chromosomes, XX, normal karyotype. A repeat amniocentesis was performed at 16

TABLE I

RESULTS OF 37 AMNIOCENTESES PERFORMED AT
SPECIFIC TIMES DURING PREGNANCY
CULTIVATED AMNIOTIC FLUID CELLS

| Gestational Weeks | Attempted | Successful | Males | Females |
|---|---|---|---|---|
| 10 | 5 | 4 | 2 | 2 |
| 16 | 4 | 3 | 1 | 2 |
| 20 | 3 | 3 | 1 | 2 |
| 24 | 6 | 4 | 3 | 1 |
| 28 | 9 | 7 | 4 | 3 |
| 32 | 8 | 4 | 3 | 1 |
| 36 | 2 | 2 | 1 | 1 |
| Total | 37 | 27 | 15 | 12 |

⋙→

FIG. 3. Cells stained with toluidine blue O. A, Normal cell derived from amniotic fluid. B, Cell derived from amniotic fluid in Case III, demonstrating metachromatic granules. C, Fibroblasts from patient with Hunter's syndrome, demonstrating metachromatic granules. D, Fibroblast derived from patient in Case III at seven days of life, demonstrating metachromatic granules.

236

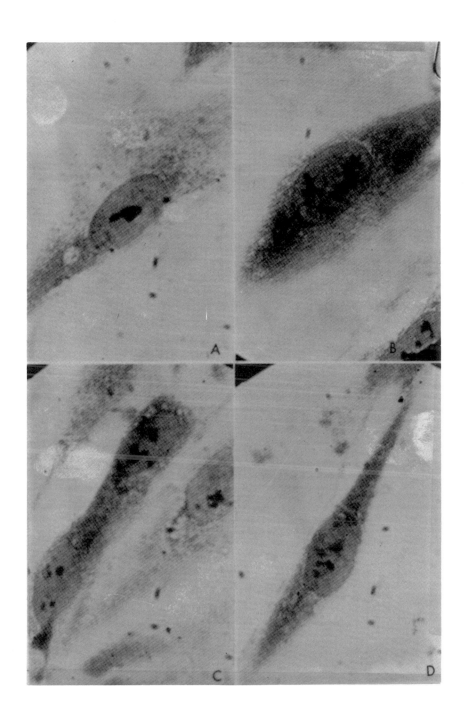

weeks of pregnancy, and again demonstrated a normal karyotype. On the basis of these findings, Mrs. S. T. elected to carry her pregnancy to term, at which time she delivered a normal, 6 lb, 11 oz female. Chromosome analysis of the baby using peripheral blood demonstrated a normal 46, XX chromosomal complement.

## Case III

Mrs. R. K., a 32-year-old female with known history of Rh incompatibility, was noted to have a rise in titer at 28 weeks of pregnancy. As part of our study, a sample of amniotic fluid was sent to our laboratory for cultivation of the cells. During growth of the primary culture, the cells were noted to be larger and more granular than normal. After the second subculture 6 weeks later, the cells were stained with toluidine blue O,[15] and metachromatic granules were noted (Fig. 3). This finding was consistent with the diagnosis of a mucopolysaccharidosis. In Figure 3 are shown a normal cultivated amniotic fluid cell, a fibroblast derived from a skin biopsy of a patient with Hunter's syndrome, a cell derived from amniotic fluid of the patient, and a fibroblast derived from skin biopsy of this patient at 1 week of age. No family history of mucopolysaccharidosis was known to the parents. At 39 weeks of pregnancy, labor was induced, and a male infant weighing 8 lb, 2 oz was delivered. Physical examination was not remarkable, but a urine examination at 7 days of life demonstrated the presence of increased mucopolysaccharide excretion using the spot test of Berry and Spinanger,[18] acid albumin turbidity test[19] (normal < .05, patient .09), and the cetyl trimethyl ammonium bromide precipitation test[20] measuring glucuronide acid content[21] (patient, 30 mg/24 hours; control, 12 mg/24 hours). Despite daily therapy with 25,000 to 50,000 units of vitamin A, by the time of the last examination at 5 months of age the patient had developed hepatosplenomegaly and bilateral inguinal hernias. Urine excretion of acid mucopolysaccharide continued to be increased, and cultivated fibroblasts derived from a skin biopsy obtained at 7 days of life demonstrated the presence of metachromatic granules.

## Case IV

Mrs. N. B., a 33-year-old Caucasian female, who had previously delivered an infant with galactosemia, developed toxemia at 33 weeks of this pregnancy. Immediately prior to elective cesarean section, a sample of amniotic fluid was obtained. Cord blood at the time of delivery had essentially no detectable galactose-1-phosphate uridyl transferase (G-1-PUT) activity (patient 0.8 μm/hour/gm Hb, normal 24.2 ± 5.0) as determined by the method of Mellman and Tedesco.[22] After 6 weeks of cultivation, the amniotic fluid cells contained no detectable galactose-1-phosphate uridyl transferase activity (normal 76.2, UDP-Gal. C[14] formed per hour per milligram total protein[15]). Mr. and Mrs. N. B. are both heterozygotes having levels of G-1-PUT of 13.6 and 9.7 μm/hour/gm Hb, respectively. The infant was immediately started on a restricted galactose diet and has continued to develop normally to the present time.

### Case V

Mrs. L. F., a 33-year-old female, had previously delivered a child who expired at 7 months of age of Pompe's disease. Mr. and Mrs. L. F. were examined and found to have reduced levels of leucocyte α-1, 4-glucosidase activity (4.3 and 3.6 μm of maltose hydrolyzed per minute per gram protein, normal 7.6 ± 1.4) as determined by the method of Nitowsky and Grunfeld.[16] Transabdominal amniocentesis was performed at 16 weeks of pregnancy and cultivated amniotic fluid cells contained normal levels of α-1, 4-glucosidase (8.3 ± 2.7 μm maltose hydrolyzed per minute per gram protein). After 40 weeks of pregnancy, Mrs. L. F. spontaneously delivered a male infant with normal leucocyte α-1, 4-glucosidase activity.

## COMMENTS

The increasing awareness of the scope of genetic disorders has made it incumbent upon physicians to provide the most precise genetic counseling possible. It would appear from this investigation and others,[12,13] that the cultivation of fetal cells obtained from amniocentesis enables the physician to establish the intra-uterine diagnosis for a number of genetic defects. Amniocentesis, although performed safely in this study and in others[13] at the end of the first trimester, should optimally be performed at 16 weeks, at which time the ease and safety of the procedure are maximal. This also allows for the processing of the sample to be completed by the end of the nineteenth week of pregnancy. Knowledge of normal patterns of enzyme distribution in cultivated amniotic fluid cells is mandatory if we are to utilize this material in a responsible manner. The normal pattern of development of a number of enzymes in cultivated fetal cells has been reported.[23] Some qualitative and quantitative differences are present at various stages of development, and caution should be exercised when any new enzyme is studied. This study focuses its attention upon the use of cultivated amniotic fluid cells for prenatal detecion. It is extremely likely that numerous genetic disorders will be capable of being diagnosed during pregnancy using either amniotic fluid, desquamated cells, or cultivation of amniotic fluid cells. The precise status of the fetus will allow for better obstetrical management of a specific pregnancy. In countries and states where therapeutic abortions are legal, this procedure would appear to be of specific value. In addition, if the modification of genetic defects is to become feasible, intra-uterine diagnosis becomes essential.

## IMPLICATIONS

The ability to precisely define the status of the fetus *in utero* should stimulate the development of new approaches for treatment and modification of genetic defects. At the present time, the treatment of genetic disorders *in utero* is limited to the management of Rh iso-immunization. Since adequate treatment or correction of many of these disorders has not been available, emphasis has been placed on prevention in the forms of genetic counseling and/or therapeutic abortion. Despite the moral, legal, and ethical questions which must be dealt with when therapeutic abortion or modification of genetic traits is considered, attempts at prenatal detection and management are warranted if we are to significantly modify the natural history of these disorders.

## SUMMARY

This study demonstrated the ability to cultivate amniotic fluid cells obtained by amniocentesis at various stages of pregnancy. Utilizing the cultivated amniotic fluid cells, the intra-uterine diagnosis of Down's syndrome, galactosemia, and mucopolysaccharidosis has been established demonstrating the usefulness of this technique for the antenatal detection of biochemical and cytogenetic abnormalities.

## REFERENCES

1. Bevis, D. C. A.: Composition of liquor amnii in haemolytic disease of newborn. J. Obstet. Gynaec. Brit. Comm., 60:244, 1953.
2. Liley, A. W.: Liquor amnii analysis in management of pregnancy complicated by rhesus sensitization. Amer. J. Obstet. Gynec., 82:1359, 1961.
3. Freda, V. J.: Rh problem in obstetrics and the new concept of its management using amniocentesis and spectrophotometric scanning of amniotic fluid. Amer. J. Obstet. Gynec., 92:341, 1965.
4. Fuchs, F., and Riis, P.: Antenatal sex determination. Nature, 177:330, 1956.
5. Shettles, L. B.: Nuclear morphology of cells in amniotic fluid in relation to sex of infant. Amer. J. Obstet. Cynec., 71:834, 1956.
6. Makowski, E. L., Prem, K. A., and Kaiser, I. H.: Detection of sex of fetuses by the incidence of sex chromatin body in nuclei of cells in amniotic fluid. Science, 123:542, 1956.
7. Serr, D. M., Sachs, L., and Danon, M.: Diagnosis of sex before birth using cells from amniotic fluid. Bull. Res. Counc. Israel, 5B:137, 1955.

8. Riis, P., and Fuchs, F.: Sex chromatin antenatal sex diagnosis. *In* Moore, K. G., ed.: The Sex Chromatin. Philadelphia: W. B. Saunders, 1966.

9. Serr, D. M., and Margolis, E.: Diagnosis of fetal sex in a sex-linked hereditary disorder. Amer. J. Obstet. Gynec., 88:230, 1964.

10. Jeffcoate, T. N. A., Fliegner, J. R. H., Russell, S. H., Davis, J. C., and Wade, A. P.: Diagnosis of adrenogenital syndrome before birth. Lancet, 2:553, 1965.

11. Fuchs, F.: Discussion of the paper by Jacobson and Barter. Amer. J. Obstet. Gynec., 99:806, 1967.

12. Steele, M. W., and Breg, W. T.: Chromosome analysis of human amniotic-fluid cells. Lancet, 1:383, 1966.

13. Jacobson, C. B., and Barter, R. H.: Intrauterine diagnosis and management of genetic defects. Amer. J. Obstet. Gynec., 99:795, 1967.

14. Harnden, D. G., and Brunton, S.: Human chromosome methodology. New York: Academic Press, p. 57, 1965.

15. Inuoye, T., Nadler, H. L., and Hsia, D. Y. Y.: A method for the assay of galactose-1-phosphate uridyl transferase in red and white cells of blood. Clin. Chim. Acta, 19:169, 1968.

16. Nitowsky, H. M., and Grunfeld, A.: Lysosomal α-glucosidase in type II glycogenesis; activity in leucocytes and cell cultures in relation to genotype. J. Lab. Clin. Med., 69:472, 1967.

17. Danes, B. S., and Bearn, A. G.: Hurler's syndrome. A genetic study in cell culture. J. Exp. Med., 123:1, 1966.

18. Berry, H. K., and Spinanger, J.: A paper spot test useful in study of Hurler's syndrome. J. Lab. Clin. Med., 55:136, 1960.

19. Dorfman, A.: Studies on the biochemistry of connective tissue. PEDIATRICS, 22:576, 1958.

20. DiFerrante, N., and Rich, C.: The determination of acid amino polysaccharide in urine. J. Lab. Clin. Med., 48:491, 1956.

21. Dische, Z.: A new specific color reaction of hexuronic acids. J. Biol. Chem., 167:189, 1947.

22. Mellman, W. J., and Tedesco, R. A.: An improved assay of erythrocyte and leucocyte galactose-1-phosphate uridyl transferase: Stabilization of the enzyme by a thiol pro-

tective reagent. J. Lab. Clin. Med., **66**:980, 1965.

23. Nadler, H. L.: Patterns of enzyme development using cultivated human fetal cells from amniotic fluid. Biochem. Genet., **2**:119, 1968.

## Acknowledgment

I thank Elvira Kavaliunas, Janet Pi, and Marilyn Swae for technical assistance, and Dr. David Y. Y. Hsia for his encouragement and critical evaluation.

# Prenatal Diagnosis of Genetic Disorders by Amniocentesis

By Gloria E. Sarto, MD.

TECHNICAL IMPROVEMENTS of cytogenetics and tissue culture, and the widespread acceptance and utilization of amniocentesis to obtain fluid for analysis allow the prenatal detection of certain inborn errors of metabolism and chromosome abnormalities. The goal of this presentation is to briefly review the work that has been done in this field and to discuss the work done at the University of Wisconsin Medical School with amniotic fluid cultures.

Amniocentesis is a procedure which has been used since the early 1930s, primarily to measure intra-amniotic fluid pressures or to treat polyhydramnios. The reports by Bevis[1] and Liley[2] on the use of amniocentesis in women with Rh isoimmunization must be credited with popularizing the technic. Major complications are: (1) perforation of placenta with feto-maternal blood transfusion resulting in maternal isoimmunization; (2) intrauterine infection with possible fetal death; (3) mechanical fetal injury, and (4) intra-amniotic hemorrhage. For several reasons an actual risk figure for these complications cannot be given; however, in the hands of experienced operators it is thought to be very small.

The amount of amniotic fluid increases with gestational age. Wagner and Fuchs[3] measured amniotic fluids in normal pregnancy: at 14 weeks, the

This investigation supported in part by National Institutes of Health grants HD00995 and HD03084 and the Racine Health Fund, Inc.

TABLE 1—*Amniotic Fluid Cell Cultures*

| Weeks Gestation | Number Cultured | Number Successful |
|---|---|---|
| <10 | 1 | 1 |
| 10–14 | 15 | 11 |
| 15–19 | 11 | 10 |
| 20–24 | 3 | 3 |
| 25–29 | 11 | 9 |
| 30–34 | 9 | 6 |
| 35–39 | 10 | 3 |

average volume of fluid was approximately 100 ml. This increased to 175 ml and 275 ml at 16 and 18 weeks respectively. The most suitable time for diagnostic amniocentesis is at about 14 to 16 weeks gestation. At this time one is more certain of obtaining amniotic fluid on a single attempt, and also one is able to have the results from the laboratory soon enough to interrupt the pregnancy should this be desired.

The cells present in amniotic fluid are of fetal origin. More than one cell type is present. There are what appear to be squamous cells, with irregular borders, which are either anucleate or have a small pyknotic nucleus. There are round or oval cells, smooth-bordered, with a larger vesicular nucleus. These may be intermediate in size with a fair amount of cytoplasm, or they may be quite small with very little cytoplasm. Both cell types may be viable. Though the total number of cells increases, the proportion of viable cells in a sample decreases with increasing gestational age.

In 1955, investigators started prenatal sex determinations based on the presence of sex chromatin in the nuclei of amniotic fluid cells. Riis and Fuchs[4] made antenatal sex determinations 20 times in 13 women, 11 of whom were carriers of hemophilia and 2 who were carriers of sex-linked muscular dystrophy. In 17 instances the prediction of sex was correct, in two it was unknown whether it was correct, and in one instance it was incorrect.

The technic for amniotic fluid cell cultures was described by Steele and Breg[5] in 1960. The various growth media they tested included Medium 199, McCoys and Diploid (GIBCO) with varying amounts of fetal calf serum. Their cultures grew only in Medium 199; however, continued investigations have shown that cells will grow in any one of the above mentioned media, if supplemented

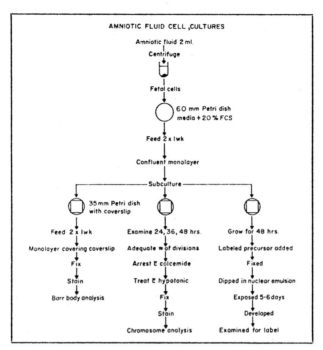

*Fig. 1—General scheme of amniotic fluid
cell culture technic.*

with adequate amounts of fetal calf serum.

Nadler[6] was the first to report on a sizeable series, when he demonstrated successful growth of amniotic fluid cells in 27 out of 37 samples obtained at various stages of pregnancy in 35 patients. Since that time, he has been successful in some 100 cases.[7]

We first attempted to culture amniotic fluid cells in December 1967.

**Materials and Methods.** Amniotic fluids were obtained from women having an amniocentesis for Rh isoimmunization and from women undergoing therapeutic abortion. Cells from 60 amniotic fluids obtained at various stages of gestation have been cultured in our laboratory (Table 1) We have had 17 failures; 7 of these were in the first 10 cultures attempted. We have found, as have others, that there is greater success with amniotic fluids obtained early in pregnancy as compared to those obtained at term. Our failures, after the technic was established, occurred with fluids which either were

246

obtained at term or were contaminated with a large number of red cells.

*Amniocentesis:* After localization of the placenta, primarily so it can be avoided when inserting the needle, the point of entry of the needle is anesthetized with a local anesthetic through the skin, fascia, and peritoneum. The needle is introduced and when it is felt that the tip is inside the uterus (the operator can feel this when he introduces the needle), fluid is aspirated. The procedure is done on an outpatient basis, takes only a short time to perform, and the patient may leave 30 minutes after the procedure is completed.

*Cell culture:* Our method of cell culture is depicted in Figure 1. If possible, 10 ml of amniotic fluid are obtained and taken to the laboratory. Aliquots of 2 ml are centrifuged at low speed (800 to 1,000 RPM) for ten minutes. The cell button is removed from the bottom of the tube, placed in a Petri dish containing F-10 medium (GIBCO) supplemented with 20% fetal calf serum and antibiotics, and then incubated at 37 C in an atmosphere of 5% $CO_2$. The cultures are examined every third day for growth; and when growth is evident, the medium is changed twice a week. When a moderate to heavy monolayer of cells has evolved, the cells are subcultured. From this stage they are treated differently, depending upon which study is to be done.

For Barr body preparations, from which the sex of the fetus can be determined, the cells are allowed to grow again until a confluent monolayer is formed, at which time they are fixed and examined for sex chromatin bodies. The presence of a heterochromatic mass on the nuclear cell membrane is generally indicative of a female sex of the fetus, while the absence of the sex chromatin mass is diagnostic of a male infant (Fig 2).

To make chromosome preparations it is best to work with cells which are actively dividing. At the appropriate time the cells are placed in colcemide to increase the number of cells in the metaphase and then processed in the usual manner.[8]

If autoradiography is to be done, the cells that have been subcultured are allowed to grow from 48 to 72 hours, are transferred into media containing radioactive precursors for an appropriate length

247

of time, and then processed for autoradiography.[8]

**Case Reports.** Using the technics described, we have been successful in making a prenatal diagnosis of (1) a male with a D/D translocation, and (2) a male fetus affected with an inborn error of metabolism, the Lesch–Nyhan syndrome.[9]

*Case 1:* A 25-year-old woman, pregnant for the first time, was 26 weeks pregnant when a chromosome abnormality, a D/D translocation, was found to exist in her husband.[10] Several possibilities existed for the fetus: (1) it could be phenotypically and chromosomally normal; (2) it could be phenotypically normal but chromosomally abnormal (as the father); and (3) it could be phenotypically and chromosomally abnormal, most probably have the $D_1$ trisomy syndrome. This condition is characterized by multiple congenital anomalies including, among others, cleft lip, cleft palate, mental retardation, deafness, polydactyly, scalp defects, eye and cardiac anomalies, and death usually within three months. An amniocentesis was performed at 26 weeks gestation. Chromosomally the infant proved to be a male and have the same abnormality as his father, a D/D translocation (Fig 3). Analysis of the chromosomes showed the presence of four D chromosomes, instead of the six which are normally present (marked by the letter D), and three 3-like chromosomes (marked with arrows) instead of two which are normally present. One of the three 3-like chromosomes is the D/D translocation chromosome; however, which one it is cannot be determined with certainty on chromosome morphology alone in all plates.

Though the infant and his father are chromosomally abnormal, they are phenotypically normal because in essence their genetic material is merely rearranged, and there is no major loss or gain of genetic material. Gross chromosome imbalance commonly results in intrauterine death; if the fetus survives to term, the infant has multiple congenital malformations. A male child, phenotypically normal, was delivered at term, which confirmed the diagnosis made prenatally.

*Case 2:* This patient was part of a large pedigree which had been studied genetically and clinically by Opitz[11] and biochemically by Salzman et al,[12] and she was a known carrier for the mutant gene causing the Lesch–Nyhan syndrome. She had been informed that her chances of having an affected child were 25%, and further, if she had a son, his chance of having the disease was 50%. Having been influenced by the fact that her mother had two sons, both unaffected, she decided to take the risk.

The Lesch–Nyhan syndrome is characterized by mental retardation, athetosis and/or spasticity and hyperuricemia, as well as self mutilation, which is probably the most distressing clinical characteristic.[13] The syndrome is transmitted as an X-linked recessive, and the affected hemizygous males lack the enzyme hypoxanthine-guanine phosphoribosyltransferase (HG-PRTase) which converts hypoxanthine to inosinic acid, a major precursor to adenine

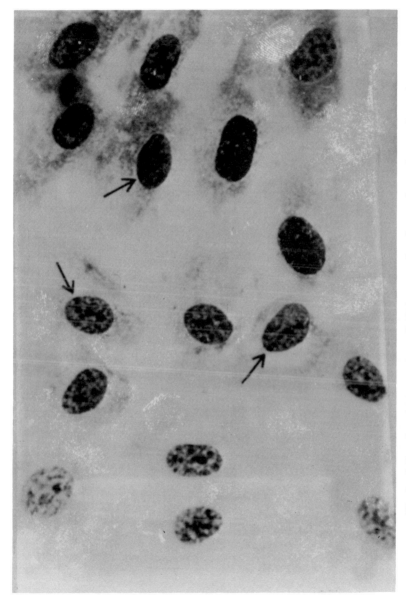

*Fig. 2—Cells cultured from amniotic fluid demonstrating the sex chromatin mass (arrows).*

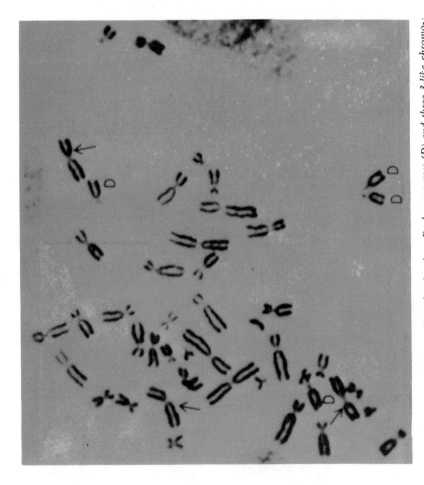

*Fig. 3—Case 1. Metaphase plate showing four D chromosomes (D) and three 3-like chromosomes (arrows). One of the three 3-like chromosomes is a D/D translocation.*

250

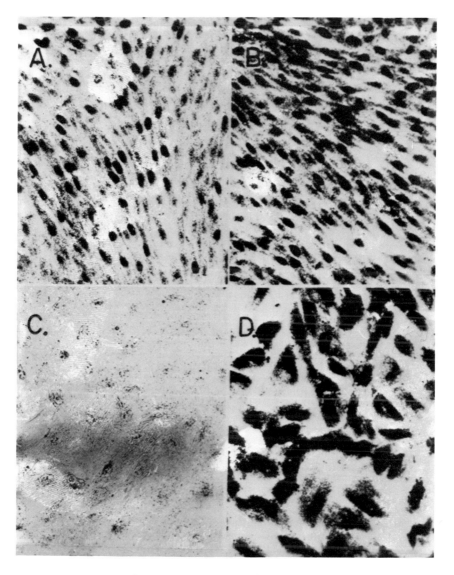

Figure 4—

A. *Control cells labeled with tritiated hypoxanthine*

B. *Control cells labeled with tritiated adenine*

C. *Patient cells labeled with tritiated hypoxanthine*

D. *Patient cells labeled with tritiated adenine*

251

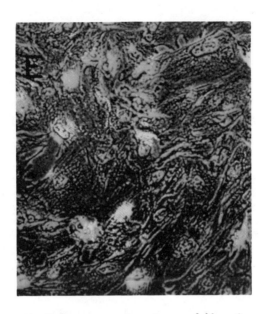

*E. Phase contrast view of same field as C, illustrating an abundance of cells.*

*All cells unstained. A, B, C, D photographed with bright field optics.*

and guanine nucleotides.[14] It has been shown by Salzman et al,[12] in cultured fibroblasts, that normal viable cells incorporate both adenine and hypoxanthine into their nucleic acids. Viable *mutant* cells, cultured from males affected with the syndrome, have adenine PRTase, but lack hypoxanthine-guanine PRTase, and are able to incorporate adenine but not hypoxanthine into nucleic acids.

At 20.5 weeks gestation a transabdominal amniocentesis was performed and the cultured cells were subjected to autoradiographic studies and sex chromatin analysis. An amniotic fluid cell culture of 18 weeks gestation was used as a control, and treated simultaneously in exactly the same manner as the patient's cell cultures. After the first subculture the cells for autoradiographic studies were divided and some were grown in medium containing tritiated hypoxanthine, while the others were cultured in medium supplemented with tritiated adenine. A second group of cover-slips with cells were used for sex chromatin studies.

No sex chromatin positive cells were found in either the control or the patient's cultures, indicating both to be male fetuses.

Figure 4 illustrates the results obtained with autoradiography. The cells cultured from the normal control patient incorporated both radioactive precursors as evidenced by the presence of reduced silver grains over the cells cultured in both types of media (Fig 4A and B). The amniotic fluid cells cultured from the patient incorporated the adenine but not the hypoxanthine as evidenced by the lack of silver grains over the cells cultured in tritiated hypoxanthine (Fig 4C). Thus the cells cultured from her were mutant; they lacked hypoxanthine-guanine phosphoribosyltransferase, necessary for the incorporation of hypoxanthine.

The patient went into labor spontaneously at 39 weeks gestation and was delivered of identical twin boys: Twin A weighing 2693 gm (5 lb, 15 oz) and Twin B 1502 gm (3 lb, 5 oz). Diagnostic studies, including elevated umbilical cord uric acid levels of 17 mg and 18 mg/100 ml respectively, and lack of the enzyme in the erythrocytes of both, proved both to be affected with the Lesch–Nyhan syndrome.

**Summary.** The use of amniotic fluid for intrauterine diagnosis of genetic disorders has been briefly reviewed and the studies done at the University of Wisconsin Medical School presented. In addition to the enzymes studied in our case of Lesch–Nyhan syndrome, several other enzymes have been demonstrated in cultivated amniotic fluid cells.[15] Future work is needed, however, to determine the "normal" levels of enzyme in the amniotic fluid cell cultures—for most of the normal levels reported have been from fibroblastic cultures, and such levels need not be normal for the amniotic cultures. This is true especially since these cultures are more epitheliod than fibroblastic. Thus, care has to be

TABLE 2—*Disorders Demonstrable in Cultured Fibroblasts*

| | |
|---|---|
| Acatalasia | Lesch–Nyhan syndrome |
| Arginosuccinicaciduria | Lipomucopolysaccharidoses |
| Chediak-Higashi syndrome | Lysosomal acid phosphatase |
| Citrullinemia | deficiency |
| Cystic fibrosis | Maple syrup urine disease |
| Cystinosis | Marfan's syndrome |
| Diabetes mellitus | Metachromatic leukodystrophy |
| Fabry's disease | Methylmalonic aciduria |
| Galactosemia | Mucopolysaccharidoses |
| Gaucher's disease | Niemann–Pick disease |
| Generalized gangliosidosis | Orotic aciduria |
| Glucose-6-phosphate dehydrogenase | Pompe's disease |
| deficiency | Progeria |
| Gout (autosomal) | Pseudoxanthoma elasticum |
| Gout (X-linked) | Refsum's disease |
| Homocystinuria | Werner's syndrome |
| I-cell disease | Xeroderma pigmentosum |
| Juvenile familial amaurotic idiocy | |

taken to determine the normal characteristics of amniotic fluid cells.

Genetic counselling up to now has had to be based on risk figures determined from the mode of inheritance of the disease: 50% chance of an affected offspring in autosomal dominant inheritance, 25% in autosomal recessive inheritance, or, as in some instances such as in chromosomal translocations, empiric risk figures ascertained from families known to have similar abnormalties have been used. A problem exists in the latter case because the risk of an abnormal child may vary widely from one family to another. In the past, some couples have elected not to take the risk quoted to them and either have had no pregnancies, or if they had a pregnancy they have sought therapeutic abortion, when indeed the fetus may have been normal. In such cases prenatal diagnosis, when successful, allows us with certainty to determine if the infant is affected. An abortion can then be sought only when the infant is known to be affected, and the risk of aborting an unaffected infant is reduced to zero.

Intrauterine treatment of certain genetic abnormalities is another new approach to therapy which prenatal detection offers. One may be able to avoid serious consequences of the disease with proper therapy instituted very early in development.

Thus, high risk patients may be selected for prenatal diagnosis. At the present time, the procedure is available to known carriers of either chromosome abnormalities or of those metabolic disorders demonstrable in tissue cultures (Table 2).[16]

#### References

1. Bevis, D. C. A.: The composition of liquor amnii in haemolytic disease of the newborn, *J Obstet Gynaec Brit Emp* 60:244–251, 1953.
2. Liley, A. W.: Liquor amnii analysis in the management of the pregnancy complicated by rhesus sensitization, *Amer J Obstet Gynec* 82:1359–1370, 1961.
3. Wagner, G., and Fuchs, F.: Volume of amniotic fluid in the first half of human pregnancy, *J Obstet Gynaec Brit Emp* 69:131, 1962.
4. Riss, P., and Fuchs, F.: "Sex chromatin in cells of amniotic fluid and antenatal sex diagnosis" in K. L. Moore (Ed.), *The Sex Chromatin*, Saunders, Philadelphia, 1966.
5. Steele, Mark W., and Breg. W. Roy: Chromosome analysis of human amniotic fluid cells, *Lancet* 1: 383:385, 1966.
6. Nadler, Henry L.: Antenatal detection of hereditary disorders, *Pediatrics* 42:912–918, 1968.
7. Nadler, Henry L.: Personal communication, 1969.
8. Yunis, J. J. (Ed): *Human Chromosome Methodology*, Academic Press, New York, 1965.
9. DeMars, R., Sarto, G., Felix, J., and Benke, P.: Lesch–Nyhan mutation: Prenatal detection with amniotic fluid cells, *Science* 164:1303–1305, 1969.
10. Doyle, Carolyn T.: Personal communication, 1969.
11. Opitz, J. M.: Personal communication, 1969.
12. Salzman, J., DeMars, R., and Benke, P.: Single-allele

expression at an X-linked hyperuricemia locus in heterozygous human cells, *Proc Nat Acad Sci* 60: 545–552, 1968.

13. Lesch, M., and Nyhan, W.: A familial disorder of uric acid metabolism and central nervous system function, *Amer J Med* 36: 561–570, 1964.

14. Seegmiller, J. E., Rosenbloom, F. M., and Kelly, W. N.: Enzyme defect associated with a sex-linked human neurological disorder and excessive purine synthesis, *Science* 155:1682–1683, 1967.

15. Nadler, H. L., and Gerbie, A. B.: Enzymes in non-cultured amniotic fluid cells, *Amer J Ob Gyn* 103: 710–712, 1969.

16. Littlefield, J. W.: Somatic cell culture in birth defects. Abstract, *Excerpta Medica International Congress Series* 191:14, 1969. □

# AUTHOR INDEX

# KEY-WORD TITLE INDEX